8 Moves to a Perfect Body

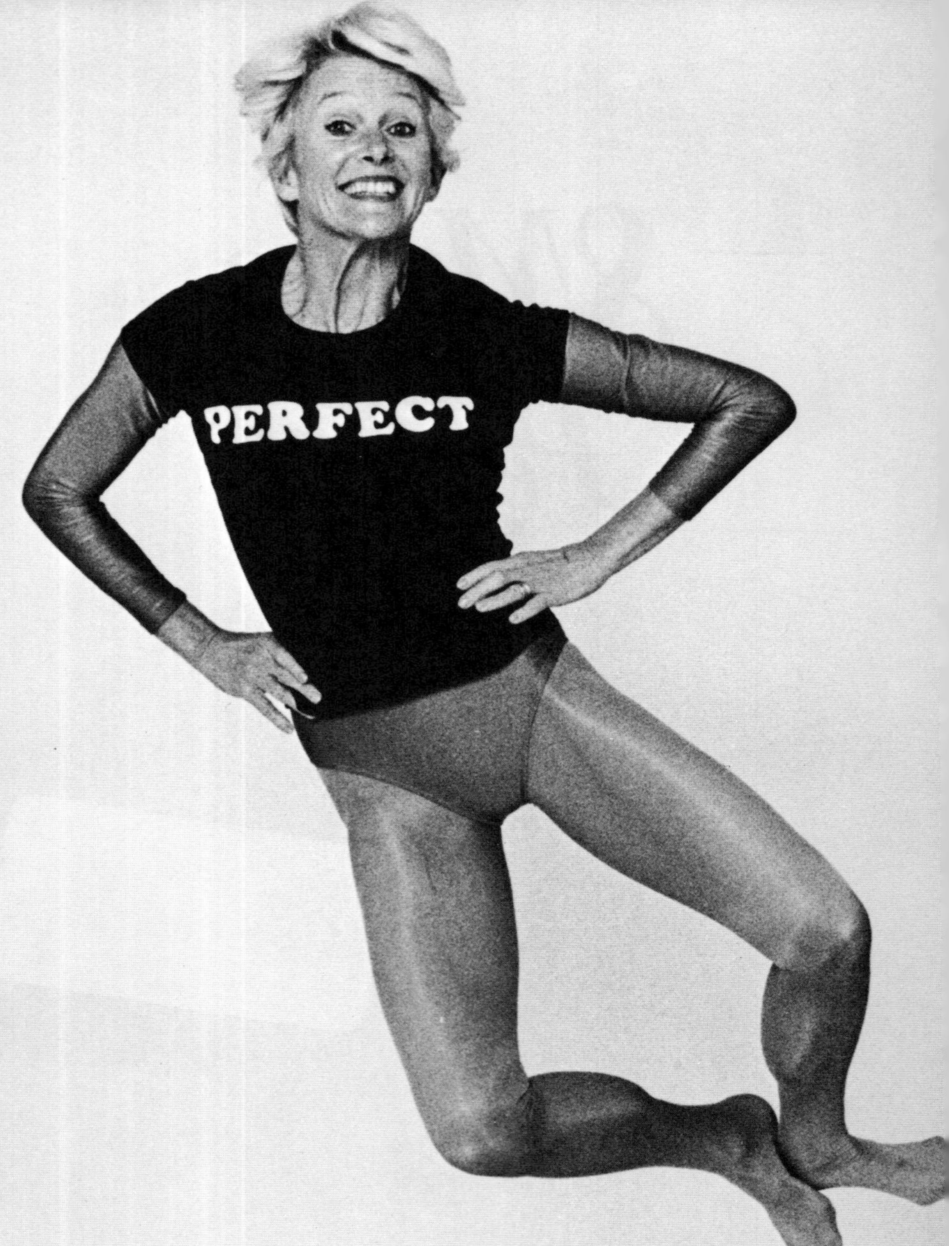
PERFECT

8 Moves to a Perfect Body

Shrink a Size in 3 Weeks without Dieting

Sheri Blair

Photographs by Lisa Berg

ACROPOLIS BOOKS LTD.

WASHINGTON, D.C.

ACROPOLIS BOOKS, LTD.
Colortone Building, 2400 17th St., N.W.
Washington, D.C. 20009

Printed in the United States of America by
COLORTONE PRESS
Creative Graphics, Inc.
Washington, D.C. 20009

Attention: Schools and Corporations
ACROPOLIS books are available at quantity discounts with bulk purchase for educational, business, or sales promotional use. For information, please write to: SPECIAL SALES DEPARTMENT, ACROPOLIS BOOKS LTD., 2400 17th ST., N.W., WASHINGTON, D.C. 20009.

Are there Acropolis Books you want but cannot find in your local stores?
You can get any Acropolis book title in print. Simply send title and retail price, plus 50 cents per copy to cover mailing and handling costs for each book desired. District of Columbia residents add applicable sales tax. Enclose check or money order only, no cash please, to: ACROPOLIS BOOKS LTD., 2400 17th ST., N.W., WASHINGTON, D.C. 20009.

Library of Congress Cataloging in Publication Data
Blair Sheri, 1936–
8 moves to a perfect body.
Includes index.
1. Reducing exercises. 2. Exercise for women.
I. Title. II. Title: Eight moves to a perfect body.
RA781.6.B57 1983 613.7'1 83-9254
ISBN 0-87491-730-1
ISBN 0-87491-727-1 (pbk.)

Cover photo: Nina Leake and Lisa Berg
Cover model: Lori Estep, *courtesy of Central Casting, Washington, D.C.*
Model for The Basic 8 Moves: Kathy Trewhitt
Art director: Christopher Jones

Acknowledgments

For my daughter,
Kelly Morrone

Special thanks to some other perfect people: The Ordway Street Olympic Team (whose fault it is), Nadia and The Sisterhood (who gave it love), Les Girls (VV Harrison, Cary Mabley and Tish Avery, who gave it fantasies), Kathy Trewhitt (who gave it youth), Lisa Berg (who gave it life); to Nina Leake, Blair Brown, Eleanor Rawson, Sophy Burnham, Kitty Kelley, Hal Bruno, Joan Gardner, Barbara Howar, Eugenie Maxwell, Sylvia Ritzenberg, Dave Roffman, Bruce Norris, Arnold Passman, and Arline Miller; to my husband, Harding (perfect torso), my mother, Belle (perfect legs), and my Aunt Alice (perfect philosophy).

***Author's note:* When you begin any vigorous new exercise program, be sure to get a medical O.K.**

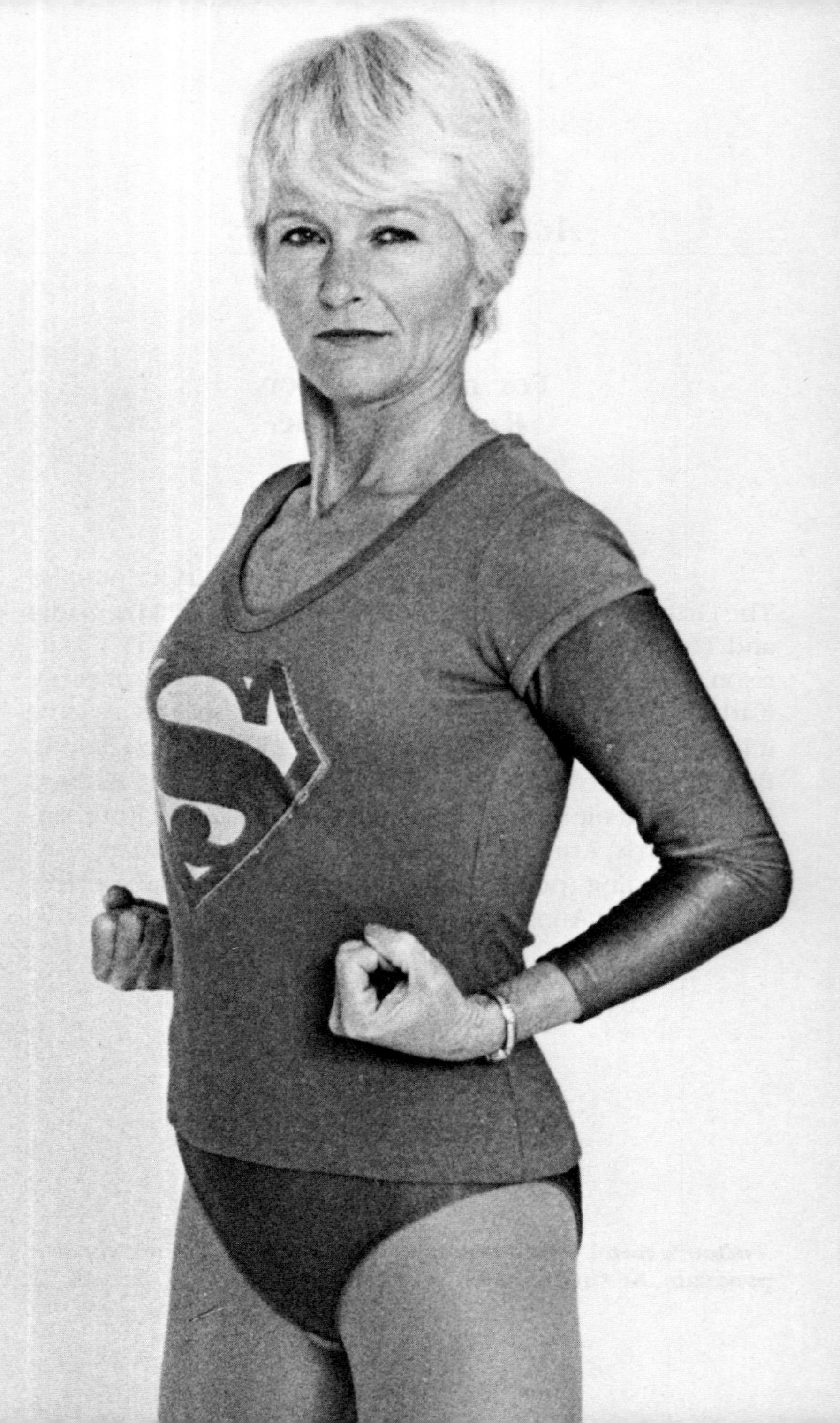

Contents

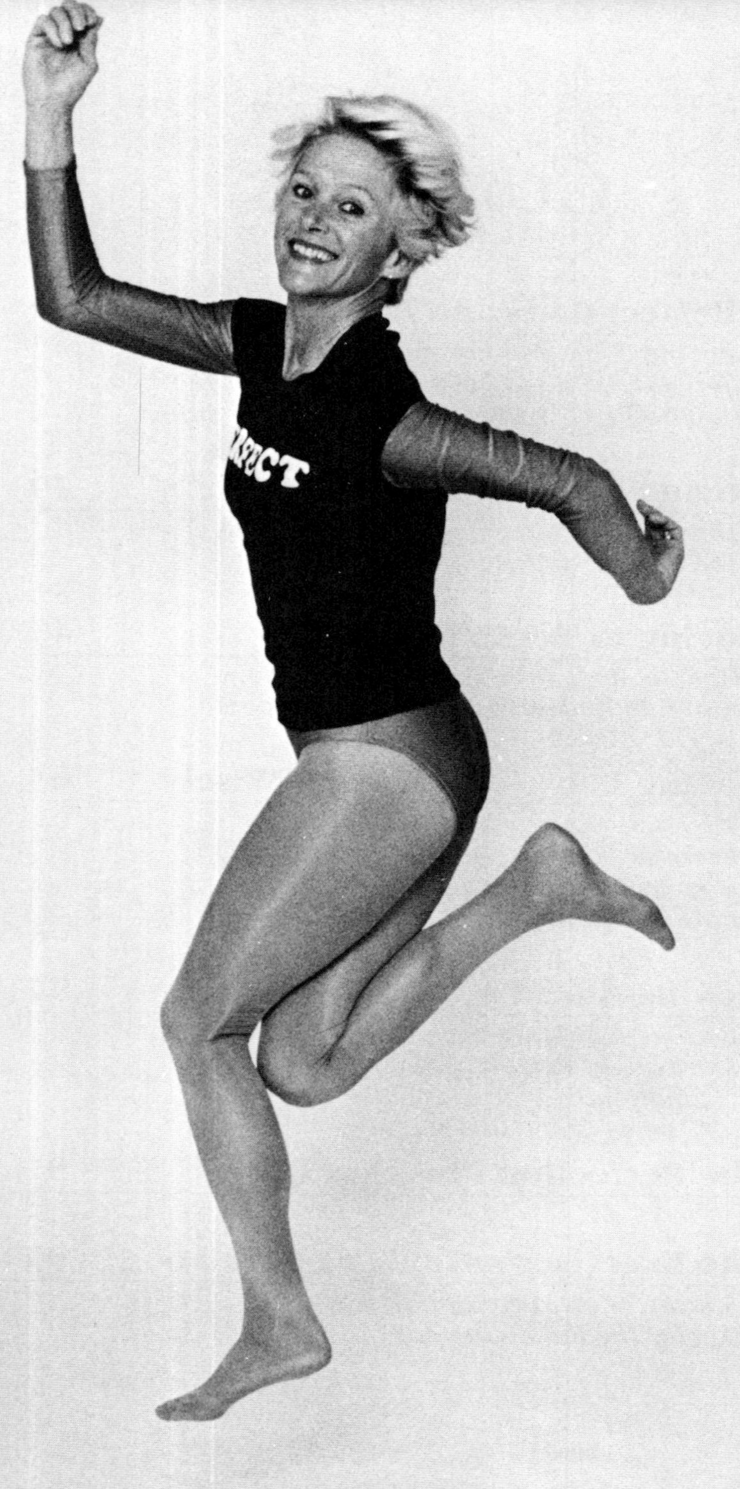

1 A Perfect Body and Peanut Butter, too

I am 47 years old and my favorite meal is peanut butter and jelly, spooned from jars.

I love junk food: Quarter Pounders with cheese, Big Wheels, sour cream and onion chips, popcorn with extra butter, Fig Newtons, chocolate chocolate-chip cones with jimmies, Goldfish, Nutter Butters, peanut butter cups, Mucho Macho Nachos, Boo Berry cereal, Pop-Tarts, fries with extra catsup, candy corn, and all the stuff left over in the trick-or-treat bowl.

I also love grownup food: Filet Mignon Bearnaise, Veal Florentine, Dover Sole Almondine, lobster, shrimp smothered in cocktail sauce, asparagus smothered with hollandaise, clams choked with buttery breadcrumbs, mushrooms stuffed with crabmeat, avocados stuffed with tuna, Cherries Jubilee, Peach Melba, and mousse au chocolat, washed down with vast reservoirs of wine.

In fact, I love *all food, anywhere*. I eat standing up in the kitchen (the spooned-in peanut butter and jelly washed down with Lancer's white); I eat sitting down at restaurants (snails, steak tartare, Caesar salad, bread, butter, and cheesecake with extra strawberry topping, washed down with champagne and Irish coffee); I eat in my car (liver sausage and Swiss on rye, extra mustard, extra mayo, washed down with a shake); I eat walking (giant pretzels washed down with Slurpees); and I eat talking (steaming Swedish meatballs, washed down with whatever I can grab from the silver tray at my elbow).

I am 5 feet 5 inches tall. I weigh the same as I did when I was 12 (115 lbs.) and my weight has stayed within the same 3–7 pound range for the last 10 years.

For the last 10 years I have been teaching exercise, 1–4 hours a day, 5 days a week.

For the last 10 years I have been wearing my perfect body.

Without dieting.

Oh, I've done my time as a Fatso. Entire other decades of time—hunched over typewriters in newspaper city rooms, hunched over bars, hunched over my obstetrician's scales (trying to pretend I'd only gained 45, not 50, pounds with my first pregnancy).

I've even been a Fat TV News Star.

It's easy to be a Fat TV News Star in Chicago. You need to wear coats most of the time there, or you scrunch down behind fake desks, or they put you in funny costumes, and cameras cut you off at the first double chin. (You've often wondered why there are so many talking heads on TV news shows?)

I've also done time dieting, in those other non-moving decades. Whatever was "in," I was on it—and I never failed (like 90 percent of the American dieting population) to regain every agonizing and depressing pound I lost.

My first meaningful effort toward my perfect body came somewhere during my mid-30s (after one of those Terrible Moments when everything south of your scalp suddenly slides toward the center of the earth with an ugly *pluggbhb* sound.)

I enrolled at Rena's Gym, where I learned a Nicholas Kounovsky-style exercise system from my personal saviour, Billy, a former gymnast: "Legs 6 inches from the floor, Sheri, not 7, SIX . . . that's it, now hold it, hold it, **HOLD IT!"**

And it was there I learned I had to make a lifetime choice: keep getting lower and larger, or *keep moving*.

What choice is there if you like to eat?

I became an exercise teacher.

*I*f you're like me—you want your peanut butter and your perfect body, too—this book is for you.

Drop that celery stick and turn that scale upside down.

From this moment on for the next three weeks, don't even *think* about weight. Don't eat any *more* than you eat now, just don't think **DIET**.

Think **SHAPE**.

Even if you're wearing a layer of mush these days, don't worry. There's a perfect body just beneath that mush, and you're about to bring it out, by turning the mush to muscle.

You are about to learn how to shrink your present body one entire clothes size in 3 weeks, without dieting. And how to bring out your own perfect body in a few more weeks—*without dieting*.

You only have to learn 8 moves, and you only have to do them once a day.

*C*lever you! You just figured out that this book is about *hard* exercise!

Of course. How else can you shrink a size in 3 weeks without starving, major surgery, or terminal stomach flu?

Of course it means a few aches along the way. (Buy an ice pack and some aspirin.)

Of course it means puffing, panting, sweat, purple-face, squashed-hair, and all those unglamorous side effects of hard exercise. (Buy a wig.)

It also means that after your very first day with this book, you're going to feel very different about yourself.

In fact, your self-esteem will shoot upwards within *five minutes* with your first move.

On the third day, somewhere in the middle of the fourth move, you may cry real tears and hate me. (Day 3 of any vigorous exercise plan is Sore City—ache to the max.)

But on the fifth day, you will be doing the whole routine with a hint of pleasure, and a *whole lot* of pride.

How the 8-Move System Works for You

The 8-Move system works like this: do all 8 Moves, in sequence, non-stop, every day for 21 days in a row. (Work *somewhat* gently if you're a beginner, ease up to full speed by day 5.)

The success of the 8-Move system comes from this combination of elements:

- There are only 8 Moves. They are not hard to memorize, and the whole routine can take less than 40 minutes a day.
- The 8 Moves strike directly at the 6 major flab-collecting areas of the body (torso/waist, stomach, buttocks, underarms, hips, thighs).
- The Moves are arranged in a sensible sequence, designed to prevent over-stress on any particular part of the body.
- The fast pace of the Moves *builds* energy rather than depletes it.

- Moving rapidly and non-stop (except for your moments with stretches and the All-Purpose Curl) burns off calories fast.
- Daily vigorous movement changes metabolism while it changes shape. For example, the Moves act almost immediately as an appetite suppressant; also, lean tissue burns calories faster than fatty tissue, so as you develop more muscle, you'll be shrinking faster even while you *sleep*.
- The 8-Move routine produces an immediate mood elevation. (Hard exercise is an emotional upper—more on this later.)
- Almost anyone in good health from 15 to 50 + (barring physical problems such as trick backs, knees, and ankles—ask your doctor before you begin!) can approximate all the Moves right away, and can work up to peak performance within 5 days.
- **After 3 weeks with the 8 Moves, a substantial amount of mush will have turned to muscle. Muscle weighs more than mush, but at this stage of development, it occupies less space.**

Exercise Teachers, Like Horses, Can Smell Fear

I can already hear the querulous, whiney little excuses hovering in the ionosphere:

"But I don't want to get muscles . . . muscles are ugly . . ."

"Isn't it dangerous to exercise from a book? I've heard that you can hurt yourself. . . ."

"I already jog (play tennis, softball, bowl, swim, etc.). . . isn't that *enough*?"

"I've tried exercising by myself. It just doesn't work . . . it's too *boring*. . . ."

Oh, hush up and listen, all of you.

First, there's no way you'll grow bulging, Rocky-esque muscles with this kind of system. It takes *pumping iron*, many hours, days, and months at a time, to get muscles that stick out. (And is *anything* uglier than molten, mottled cascades of *mush*?)

Second, it is highly unlikely you'll hurt yourself working out with a book. A book doesn't shout at you like a boot camp sergeant, or snicker behind your back if you miss a beat. Nor does it exert competitive pressure that may lead you to over-exert.

Besides, if you *don't* "hurt" (feel what I call the "ache-and shake") while you're exercising, you know you're not allowing your muscles to do their best. Ache-and-shake is a harmless and temporary chemical reaction to deep muscular exertion. If it becomes unbearable, just stop for a few seconds until it goes away, then push onward and don't worry about it.

Third, no popular sport, (and I include jogging and swimming), is enough for the whole body. Legs and arms get some attention from these sports, but they do almost nothing for your abdominal muscles, and stomachs stay just where they are. Down. Or out.

Finally, exercise is only boring if it's too easy. It's never boring if it challenges you—and I can assure you, the 8-Move system is challenging.

Here are a few tricks to use to psych yourself up:

Trick 1: Let's Play Fantasy

Pretend you're 12 again. When you were 12, what did you dream of being when you grew up?

When I was 12, I wanted to be a woman warrior. I saw myself as a lean, bold Viking Queen, by day sheathed in silver chain mail, leading endless armies of adoring men into battle; by night sheathed in silver lamé, luring select worshipping generals into my tent . . . .

So, I psych myself into my "solo" workout by wearing a Superman T-shirt, listening to march music, and thinking, "Conquer!"

Then there's a man I know who always wanted to be a toreador.

To ready himself for a workout, he clicks his heels, raises his chin, looks sideways through slit eyes, puffs out his chest, curls his lip into a sneer and shouts, "Ha! Toro!" Then, since he doesn't own a cape or skintight black pants, he dons a sweatsuit and turns his favorite flamenco tape up to OLÉ!

Another friend is the perpetual star of a perpetual Broadway hit musical. Her ritual: black tights, shiny silver leotard, lots of makeup, and the cast album of "A Chorus Line."

Come on, *think* back. Stare into your memory. Were you Tarzana, Queen of the Jungle, or Cleopatra, Queen of the Nile? Were you Wonderwoman? Miss America? A Las Vegas showgirl or a Gibson girl? A Charlie's Angel or a Hell's Angel? Chris Evert Lloyd in white shorts or a stripper in black mesh stockings? The lady bareback rider or the girl on the flying trapeze?

Think back to your perfect fantasy body in all its costumed splendor. Play back the majestic music that suited it—and move!

Trick 2: Let's Play Sculptor

Mold your perfect body (or perfect body-to-be) with your hands.

This means staring at your *real* self in a *real* mirror, stark naked if you can stand it.

Two things will happen automatically.

First, you'll stand up straight. Then you'll suck your stomach in. See? A large portion of mush is halfway gone.

Still more paunch? Grab the skin above your diaphragm and tuck it under your rib cage. Love handles around the waist? Grab with both hands and push them behind your back. Hips a little puffy? Shove as many of *those* layers as you can behind your back.

Pouches on the inner thighs? Cross one leg behind the other and squish until they disappear.

Now turn around and look over your shoulder. Puckers in the upper thigh? (*Yuck*. Lips may be puckered; upper thighs, never.)

Grab that sagging derriere and *hoist*.

You've got the message.

If your posture and your hands can correct some mush temporarily, just think what **permanent muscle** could do.

Trick 3: Let's Pick the Right Moving Space

You'll need about 6 feet by 8 feet, or 7 feet by 7 feet, preferably carpeted. When you choose this space, forget that it's a slice of bedroom or living room, office or kitchen. Once you start your daily Moves, it becomes a gym and nothing else.

Trick 4: Let's Pick the Right Moving Time

Don't sit around and wait until the "spirit" moves you. Set aside a specific time of day (when your stomach is empty), mark your 3-week (or 8-week) schedule in your calendar and *stick to it*.

Helpful hint: I have 3 favorite times: morning, so I can get it over with and because it wakes me up fast; pre-lunch, so I have less appetite; and late afternoon, because it kills the blahs, blocks the urge to nibble or nap, and gives me a new blast of energy for the evening's fun and games.

The final trick: remember your goal. Repeat out loud: **Three weeks from now I will be one size smaller**. I may weigh the same (because muscle weighs more than mush), but I will be one size smaller.

What else do you need before you start to move?

A testimonial!

Consider the back cover of this book. Me.

Every August I collapse into a lounge chair at the beach and move nothing except my right hand, which brings junk food and frozen daiquiris from table to mouth. Every Christmas-time my classes stop for two weeks and I collapse into the cranberry sauce, the pecan pie, and the eggnog.

Yes, twice a year *I* have to shrink a size. And I *refuse* to diet.

Remember, at 47 I'm hardly your world-class ingenue. So if I can do it, so can you. Turn on your music, turn the page, and go!

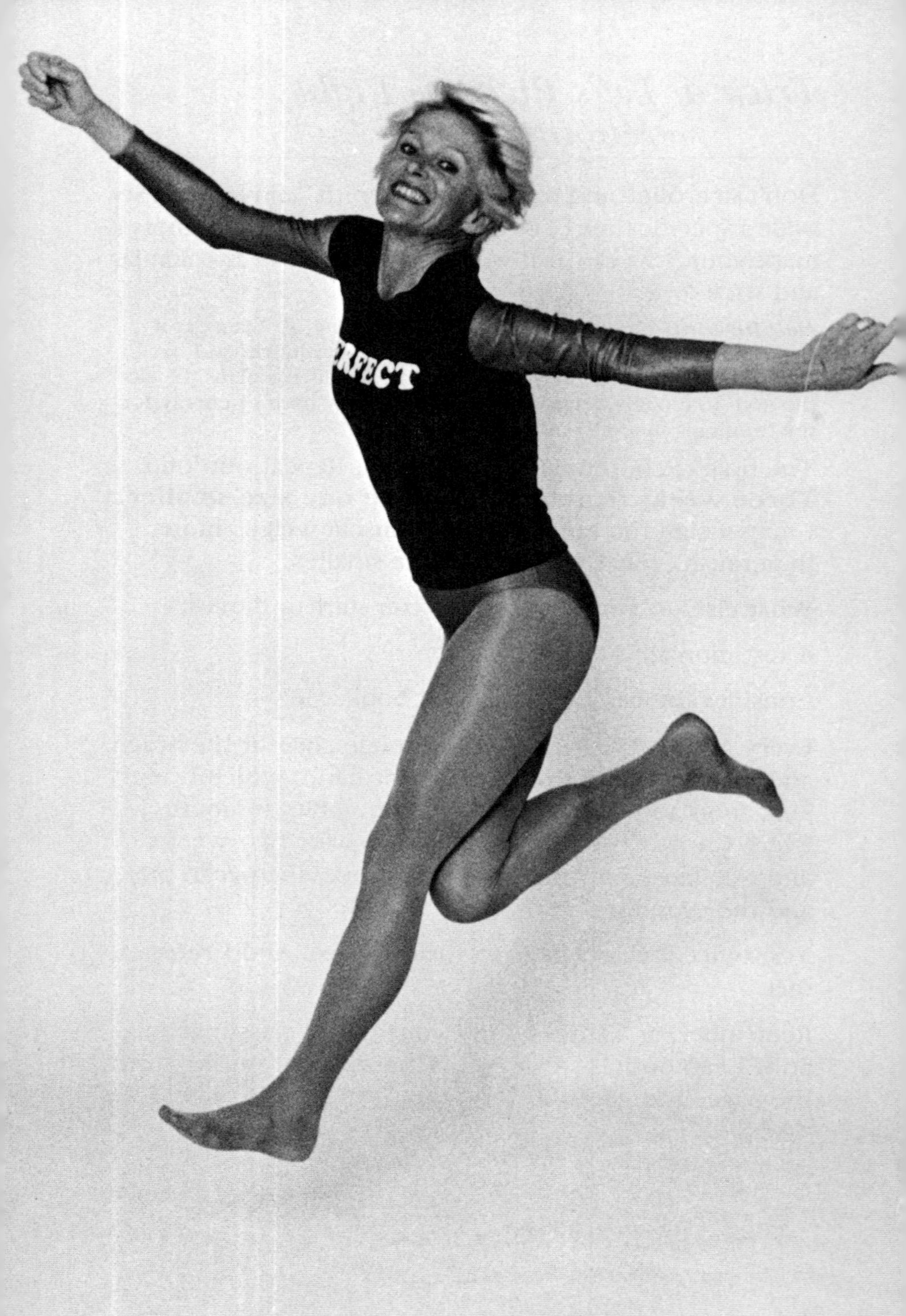
ERFECT

2 *Moving Faster—Getting Smaller*

Your first move is *up*—into The Big Leap!

Your goals in this Move: cardio-vascular endurance, tightening mush from thigh to toe on the fronts and backs of your legs, maximum calorie-burn, and energy for the next 7 moves.

The first 5 minutes of this move also serves as your warmup for the whole routine.

Your breathing: In and out. Never hold your breath. Scream if necessary, but don't stop breathing.

Your suggested music (in case your fantasy music is out of print): "Hooked on Classics I and II," RCA. Start out with Side 2 of Classics I, Tchaikovsky, etc. Stick with a superfast beat.

Alternatives for this move: a *very brisk* 1 hour, 15 minute walk. If you're a runner, try 2 to 2½ miles. And if you jump rope the true-blue schoolkid way (both feet off the ground, continuous hopping), about 12 minutes will do.

Helpful Hint: If you don't have a cushiony rug, wear running shoes for this Move, and build your endurance from 10 to 25 minutes within 5 days.

1 *The Big Leap*

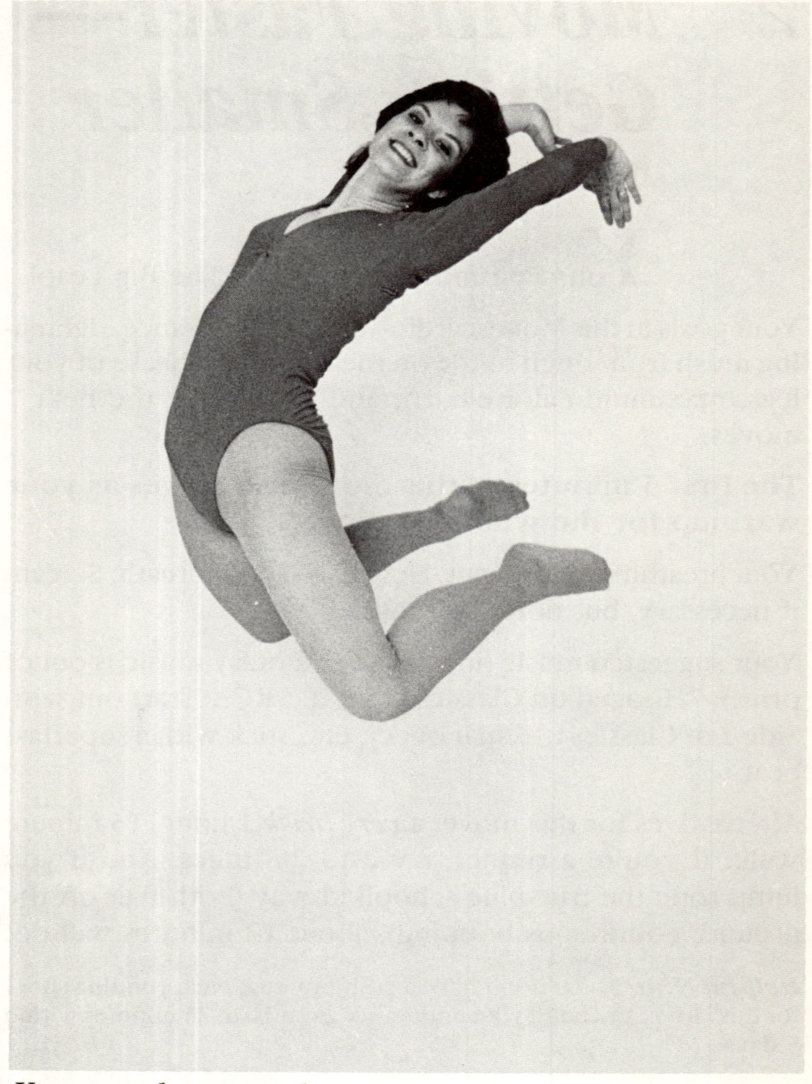

Up, up and awa-a-ay!
Get those feet off the floor for 25 minutes, ***nonstop***.

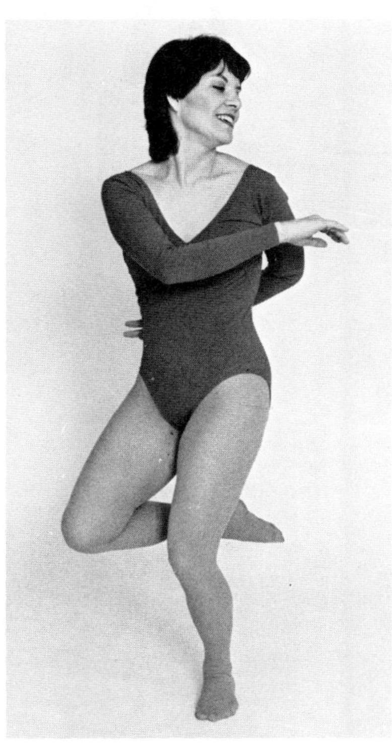

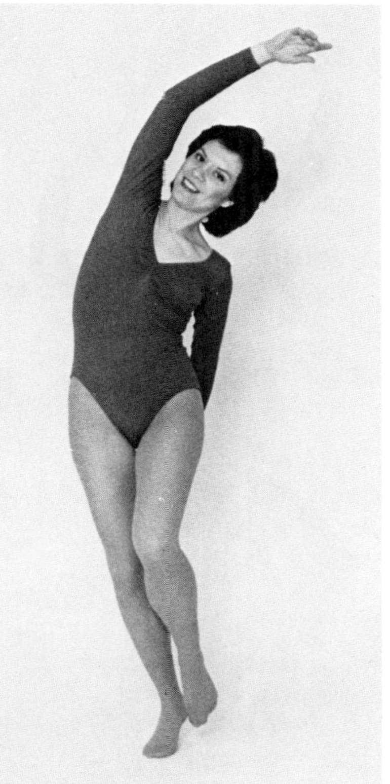

Low Gear: *(5 minutes) Warm up and loosen up with 5 minutes of easy, sloppy jogging around your space, landing with knees slightly bent, rolling from the ball of each foot to the whole foot. As you jog, bunch your shoulders and relax them, roll your head around and begin to use your arms.*

Swing them from front to back, side to side. Stretch toward the ceiling, one arm at a time. Fling both arms first to one side, then the other. Now keep them swinging with the beat of your feet.

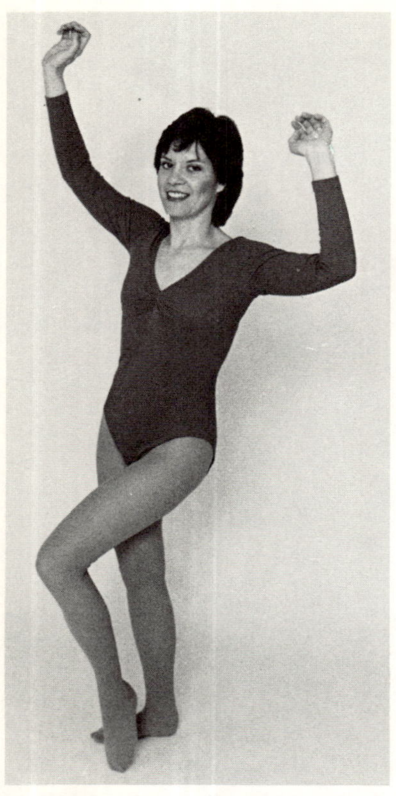

Second Gear: *(8 minutes); Dance! Spend 2 minutes with the dances (and imaginary partners?) of your choice: Disco. . . country. . . samba. . . rock!*

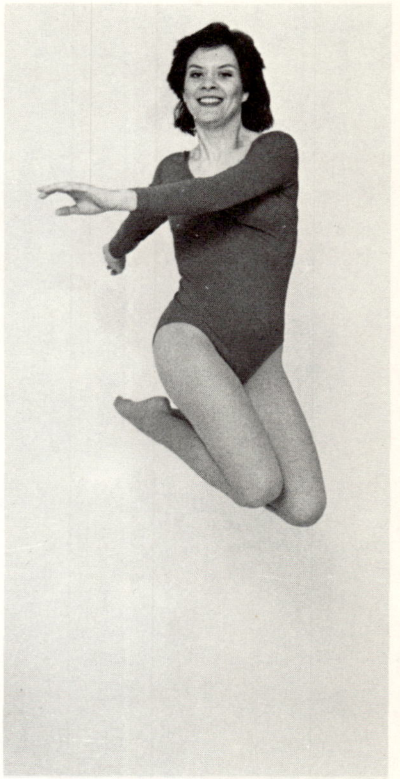

Move back to the 50s for 2 minutes of the Twist, Chubby Checker style.

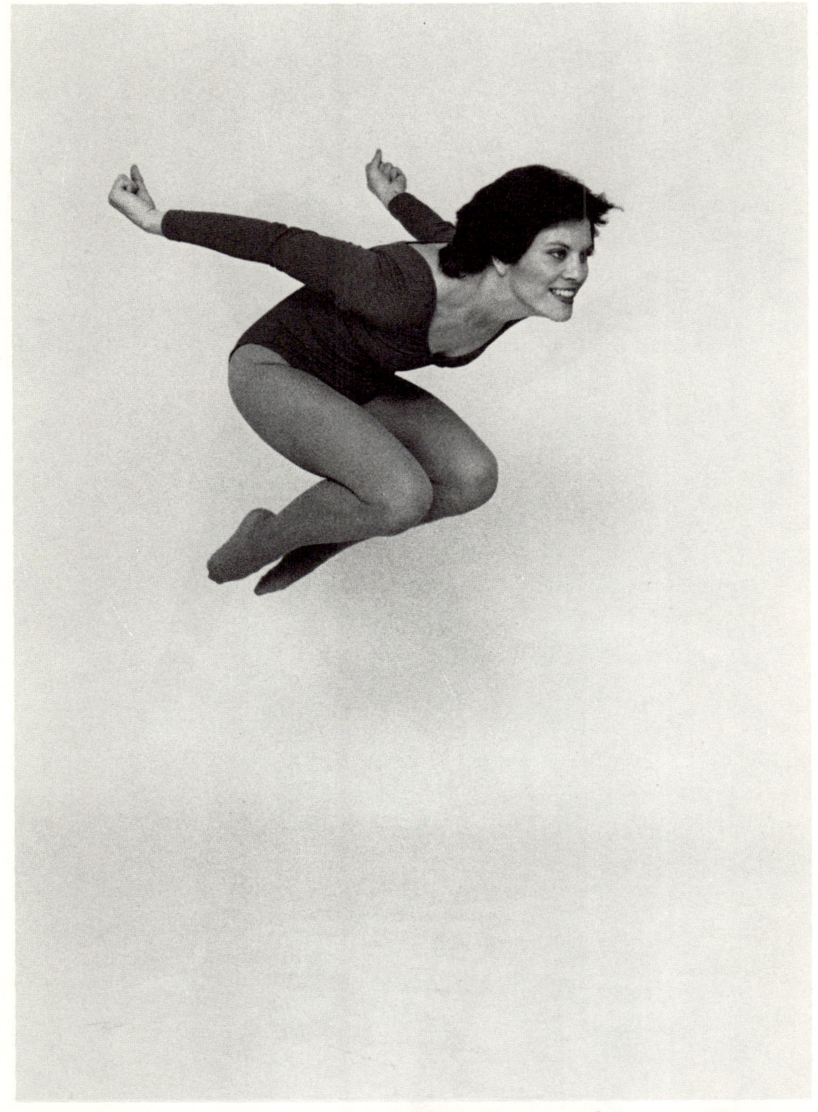

Move back another decade for 2 minutes of Bunny Hops.

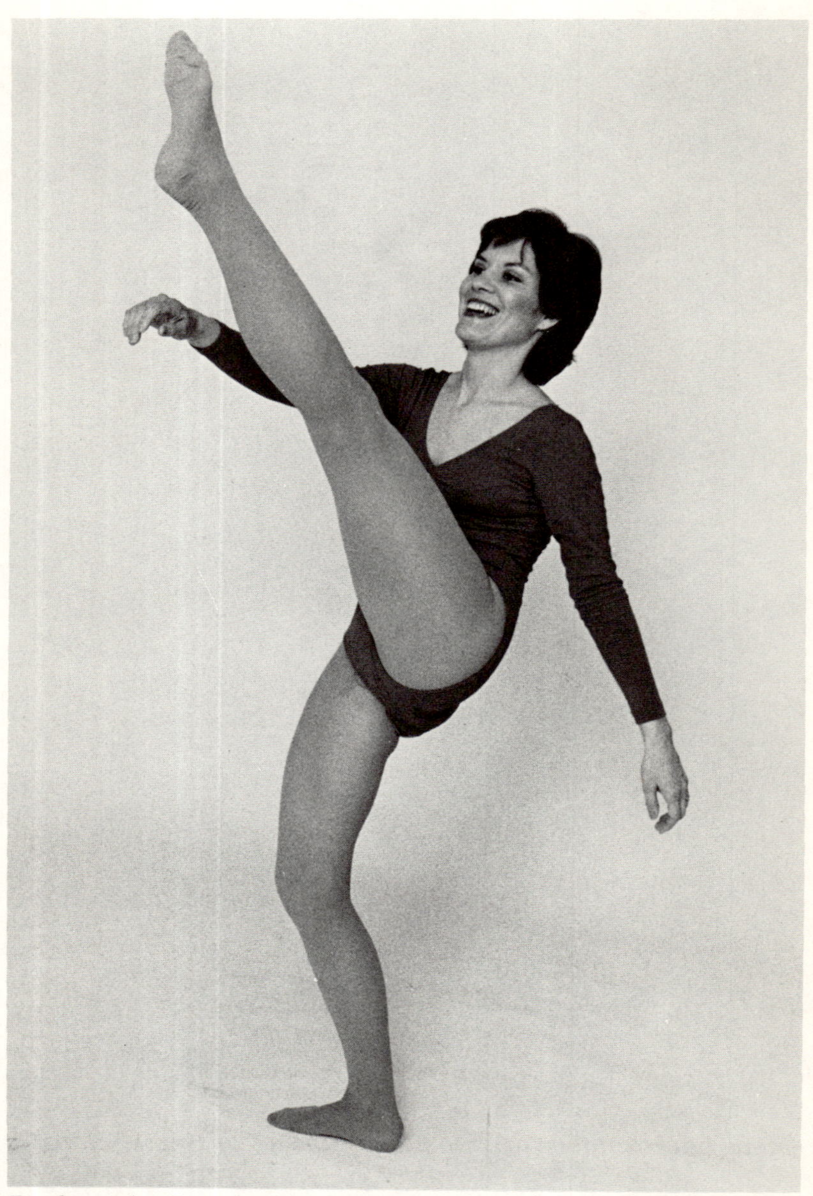

Back to the Roaring 20s for 2 minutes of the Charleston!

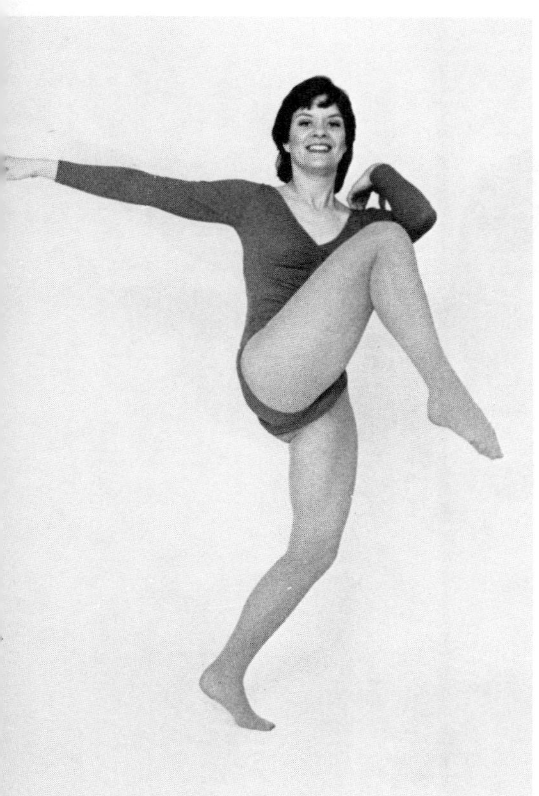

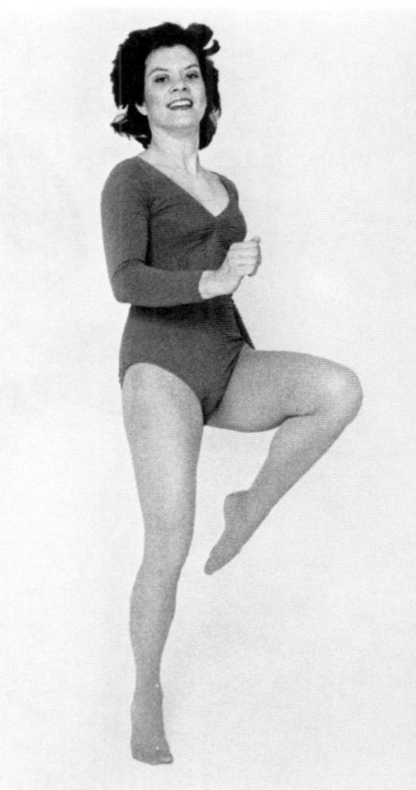

***High Gear:** (7 minutes): Spectacular action! Start with a 2-minute strut, leading that jazz band down Bourbon Street. Bored?*

Feed in 1 minute of Rockette knee lifts, alternating knees. Backs of legs aching and shaking? Good! Applause!

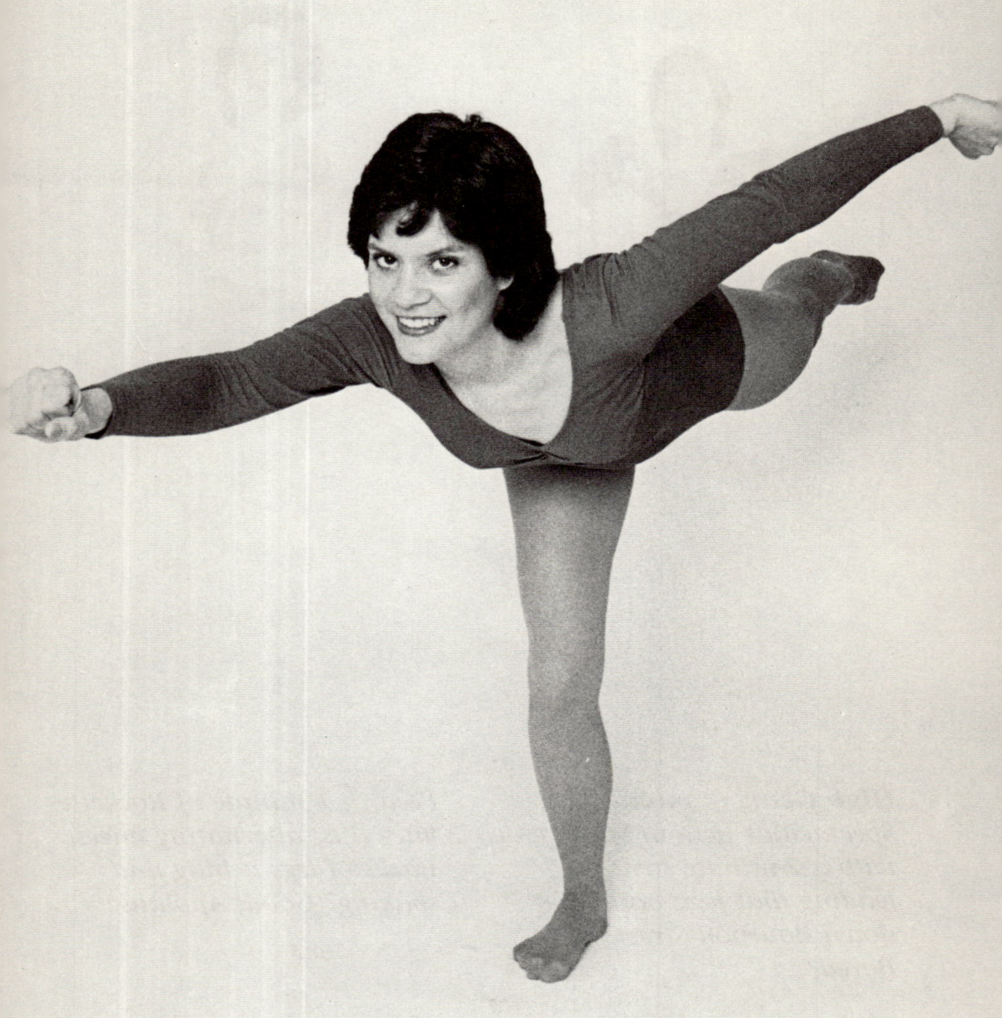

Attack fronts of legs with a minute's worth of Broadway-style lunges, leaning forward and kicking legs up behind you. Encore!

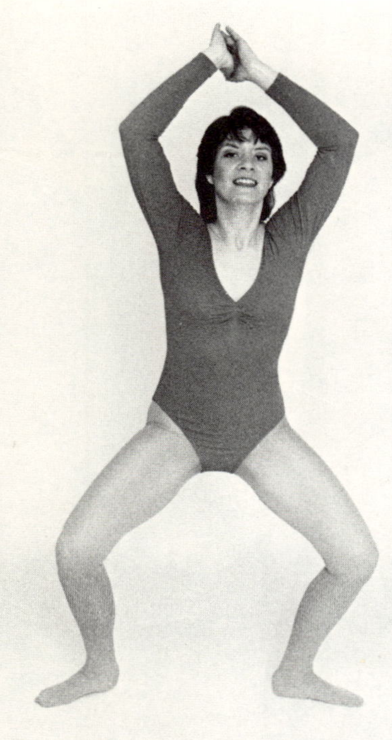

Time for 2 minutes of boot camp jumping jacks! Snap those feet apart, soldier!

Note: **The world's record for nonstop jumping jacks is only 27,000. Beat it!**

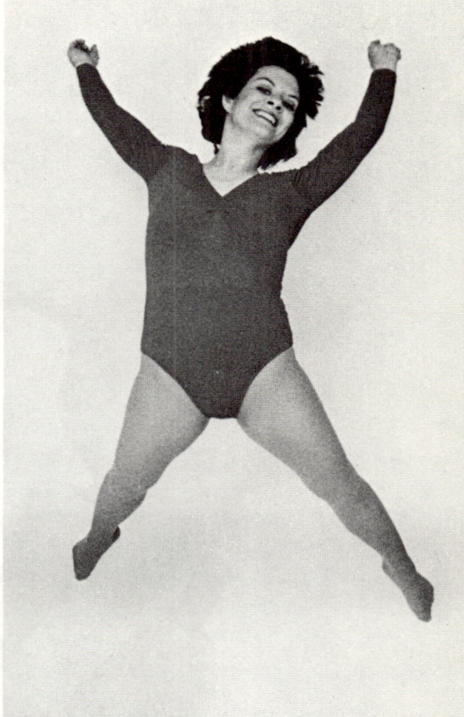

Wheezing? Snorting for breath? **Hooray!** *Not much time left in the game and the crowd is going wild! Give them a full minute's worth of your best high school cheers!* ***Go, Team, Go!***

Gear Down: *(5 minutes) Ease back again, first to your sloppy jog, then to a march, then to a last-minute walk. Let your breathing subside. Stop. Shake out each leg. Massage your leg muscles with your hands, and*

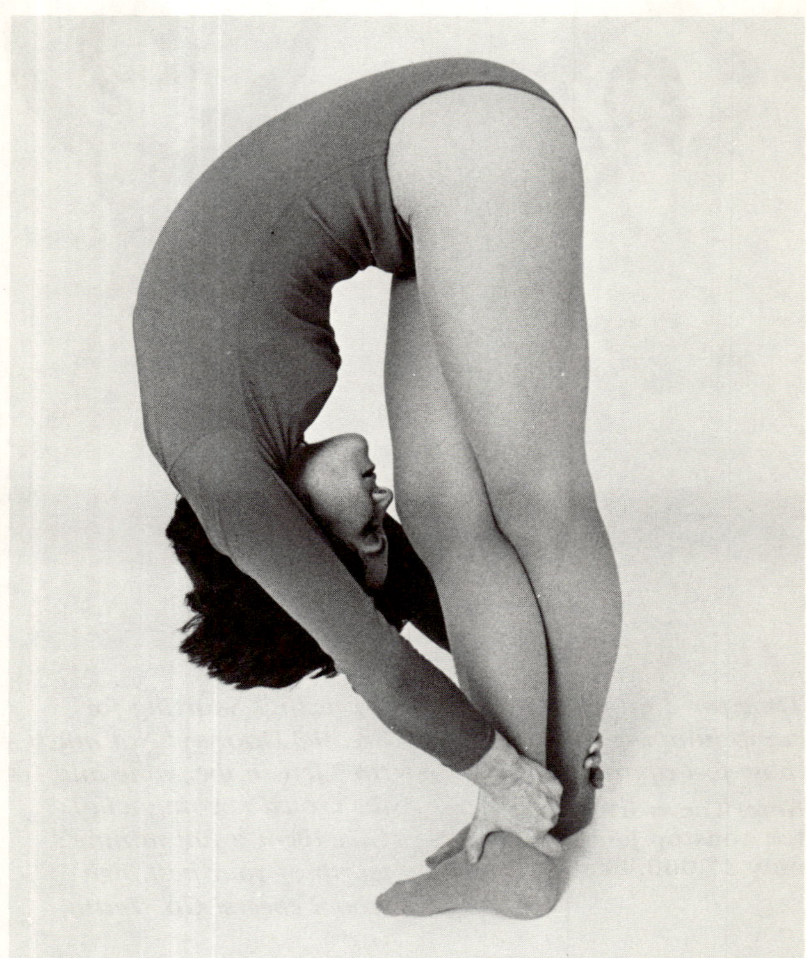

Stretc-c-h-h out with the Runner's Classic. Cross one foot in front of the other. Keep both knees straight, lean forward slowly, grab your ankles and hold your nose as close to your knees as possible for a slow count of 10. Reverse leg positions and repeat.

Okay, end of rest period. On to the rest of your body.

Your goals for the next 7 Moves: to assault and shrink every remaining pocket of mush.

Your breathing: there's a continuing argument within exercise physiology circles whether to exhale or inhale at the maximum exertion (ache-and-shake) point of an exercise.

I say do what feels better and never hold your breath. Sob, sing, shout nasty epithets at me. Just keep breathing.

Suggested music (again, in case your fantasy music is unavailable): "Booked on Broadway," Polygram Records. Pace for all 7 moves: peppy medium fast.

Alternatives: *NONE.* My exercises are the best.

Helpful hint: Muscles you didn't know you had will be sore for the first five days. Smile—you're shrinking. More about aches and pains in Chapter 4.

2 *The Waist-Cincher Stretch*

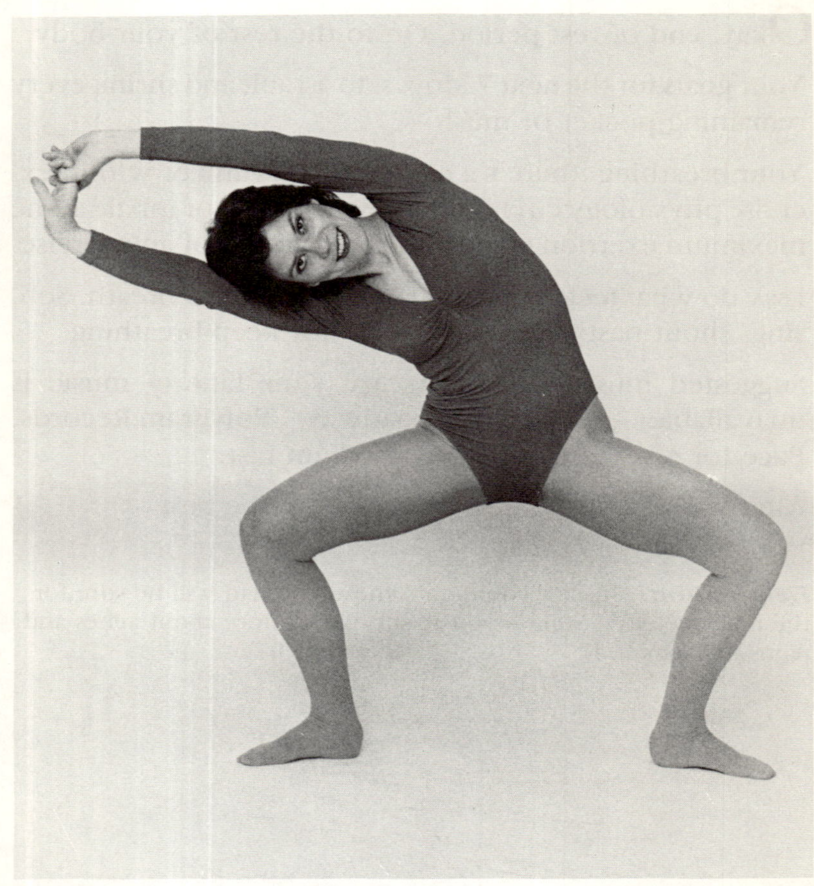

Stand with your feet about 2½ feet apart. Bend knees and push pelvis forward. Grab your left hand with your right hand and bend sideways from the waist, keeping left arm ***directly*** *over your left ear. Now* ***PULL*** *your upper arm sideways as hard as you can.*

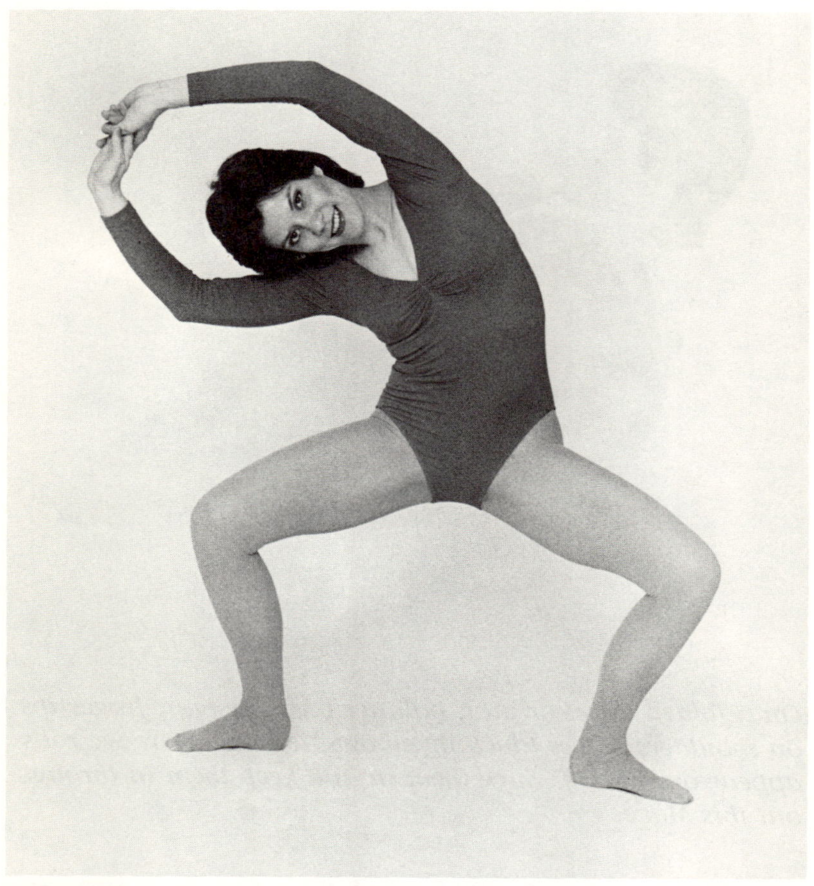

***RELAX** and bend arms **without** raising your torso. This is 1 repetition. Repeat at a brisk pace, 30 times pulling right. 30 times left. Sides of waist and torso aching and shaking? Good.*

Note: **History's smallest waist, 15 inches, belonged to Catherine de Medici (1519–1589). Yours can be smaller.**

3 *The Balanced Paunch-Puncher Pullup*

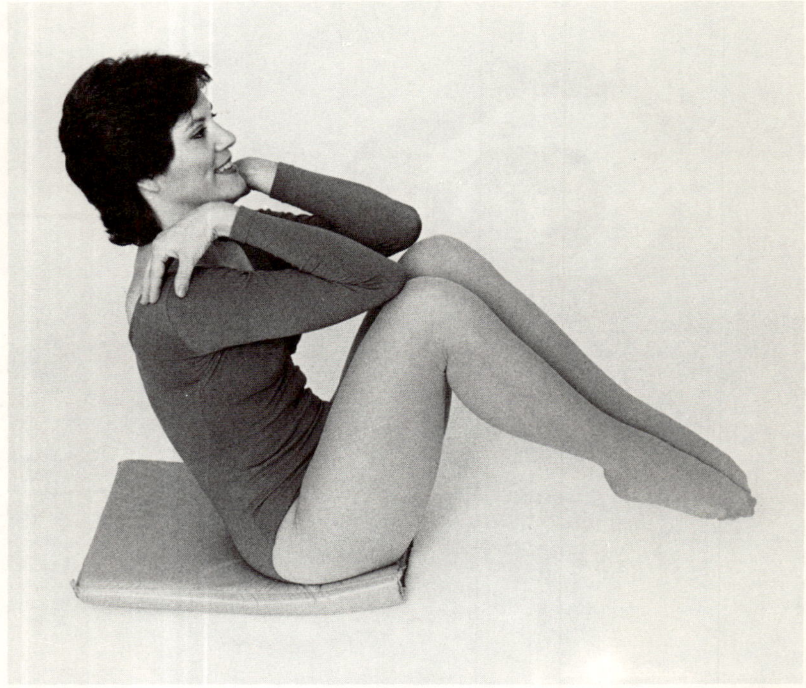

On a folded towel or mat, balance on your rear, fingertips on shoulders, knees touching elbows, legs together. See rolls appear on midriff? Suck them in and keep them in throughout this Move.

Note: **In 1964, John Greenshields, a 28-year-old ex-FBI agent, did 14,000 situps in a row in 6 hours and 10 minutes. You can do better.**

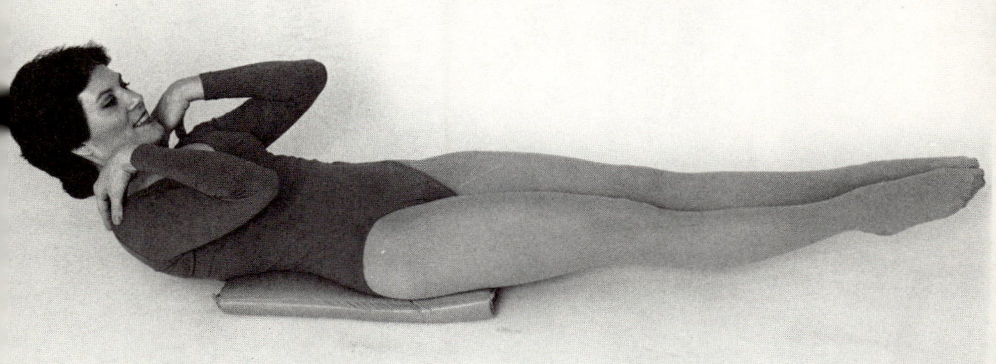

Now straighten your legs and lower them to 6 inches from the floor, while lowering your upper body until the small of your back touches the floor.

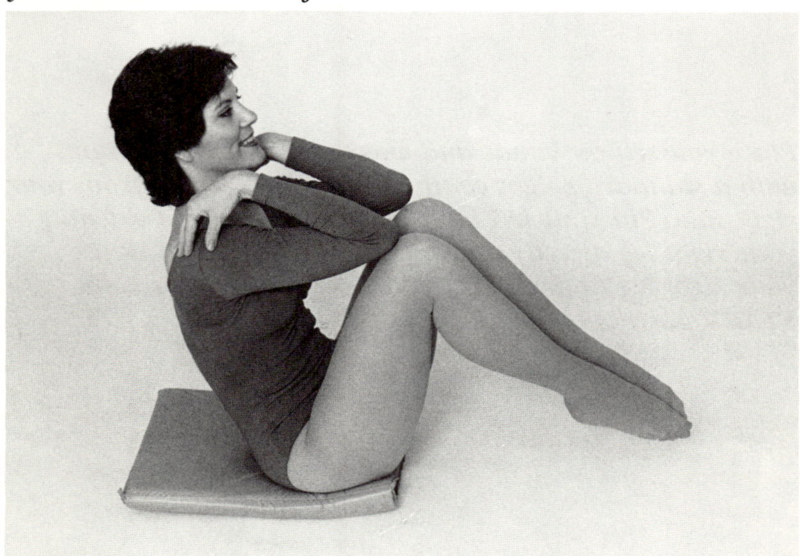

Pull elbows and knees together again. 30 repetitions. Feel the ache-and-shake beneath the midriff mush? Right on target!

4 The Honed-Down Hip Lift

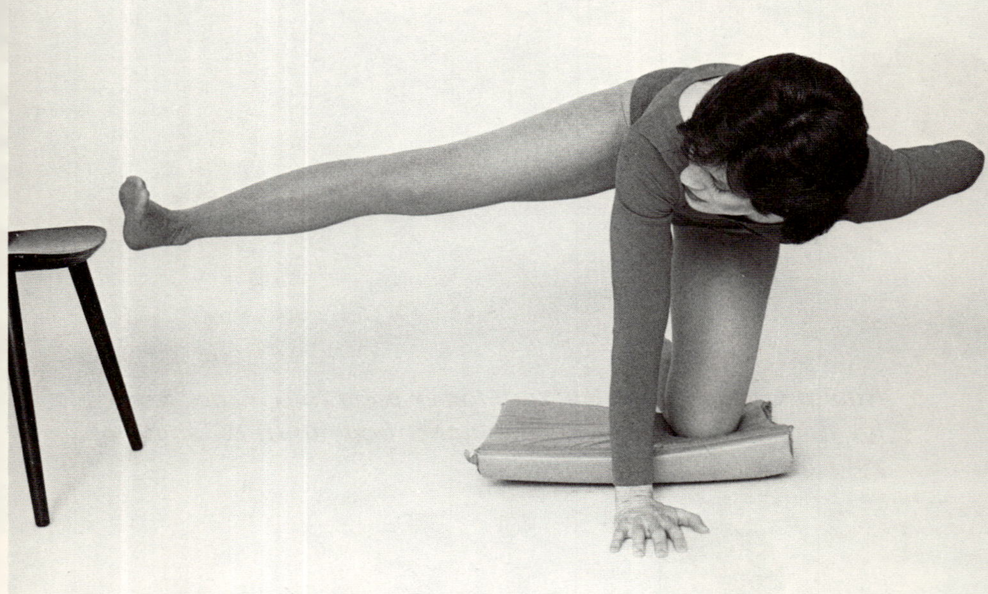

Place yourself on hands and knees on an extra cushion, with a standard-height chair about a leg's length from your right side. Put your left hand on your waist and extend your right leg directly out to the side, foot flexed. Raise your right leg to the height of the chair seat. This is the ***START*** *position.*

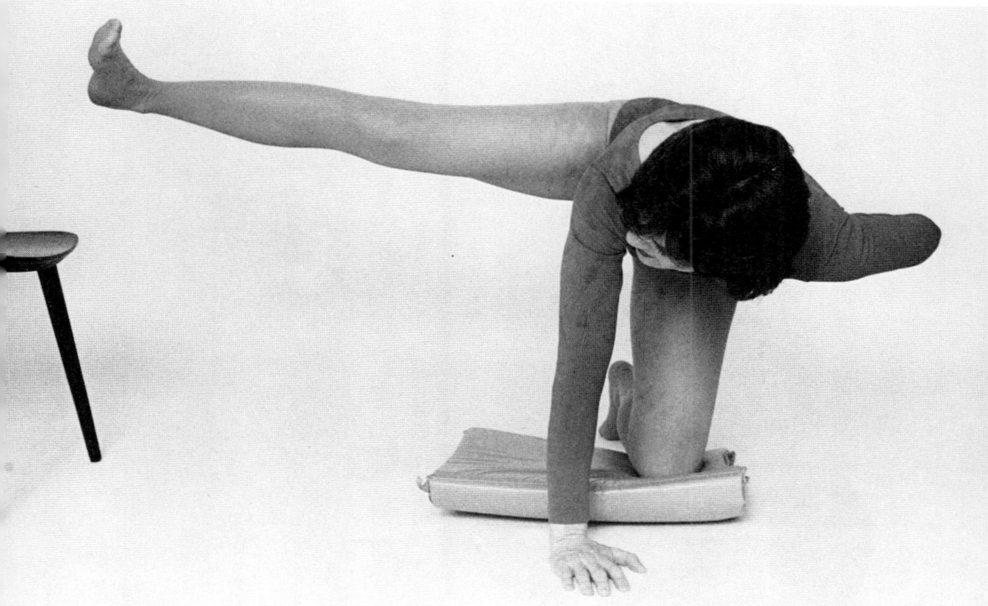

*Now **LIFT** that leg **as much higher as you can** (6 inches? 8 inches? 12 inches?) and lower it to **START**. 30 repetitions with right leg extended, 30 with left leg.*

This move is known among my students as "the smoking hip."

Helpful hint: If you can't reach *START* for starters, start at the floor and work up.

5 *The Legs-Up Diaphragm-Slam*

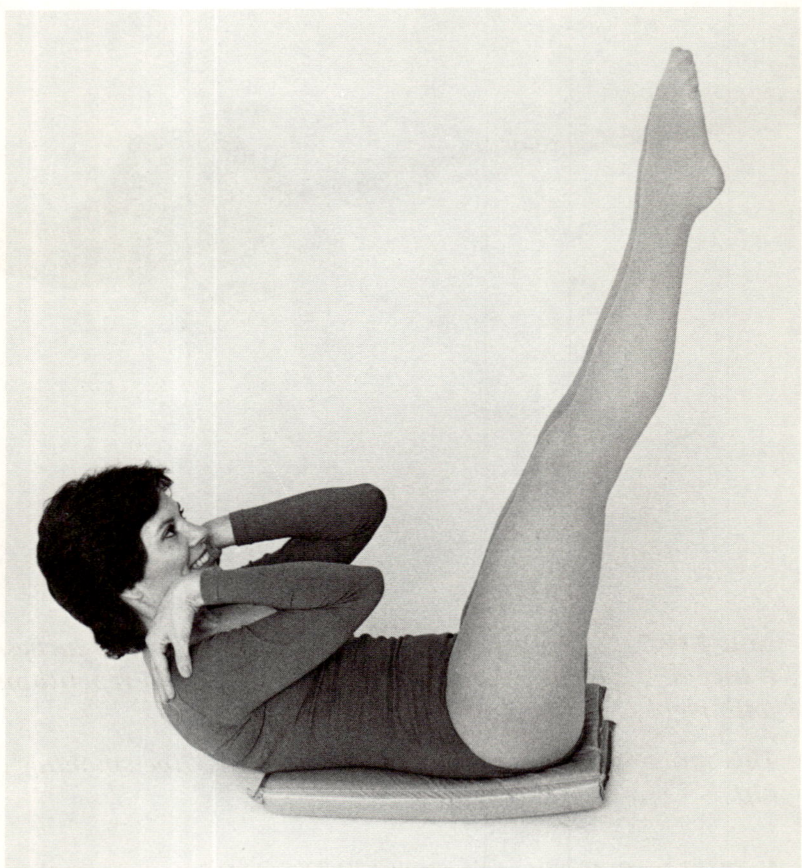

Lie with your back on your cushion, legs together, toes pointed at the ceiling, fingertips on shoulders and elbows pointed at knees. (Keep elbows pointed at knees at all times! No throwing shoulders, arms or head forward! Cheating! Straining the wrong muscles!)

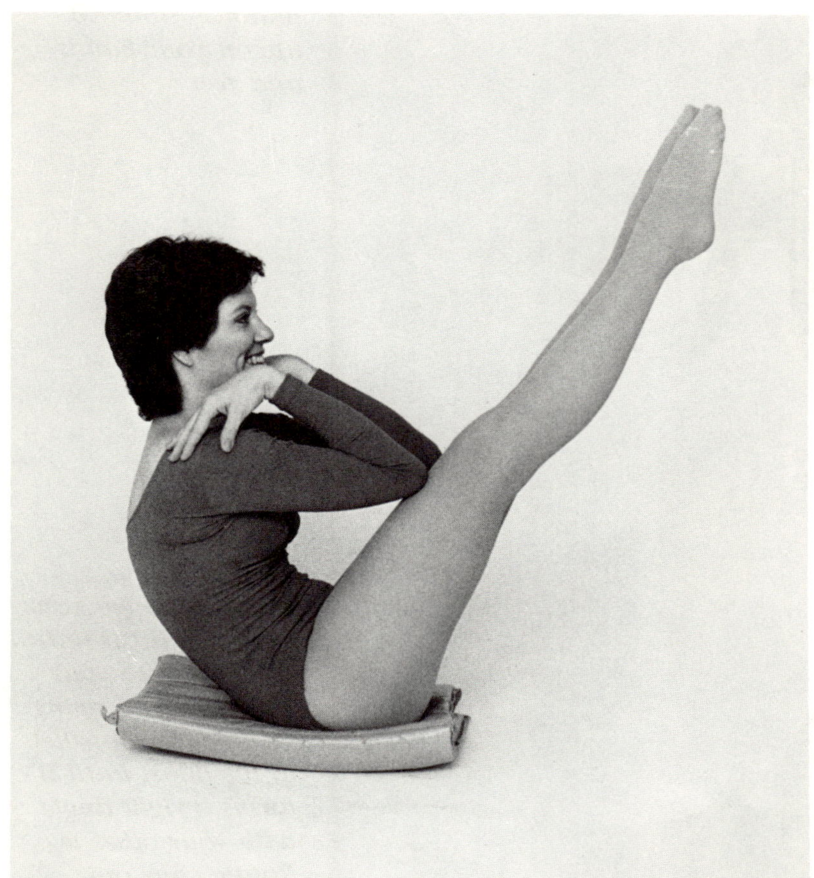

Using ***only*** *your stomach and diaphragm muscles (where the shake-and-ache will hit like a jackhammer), lift your torso until your elbows touch your knees. If you can't actually touch those knees, don't panic. Approximate it. It's the* ***effort*** *that counts, and your diaphragm will thank you. Raise and lower torso 30 times, building up from 15 repetitions.* ***Note:*** **World's record for consecutive situps without feet pinned: 26,000. Go for 26,030.**

6 *The High Thigh Push*

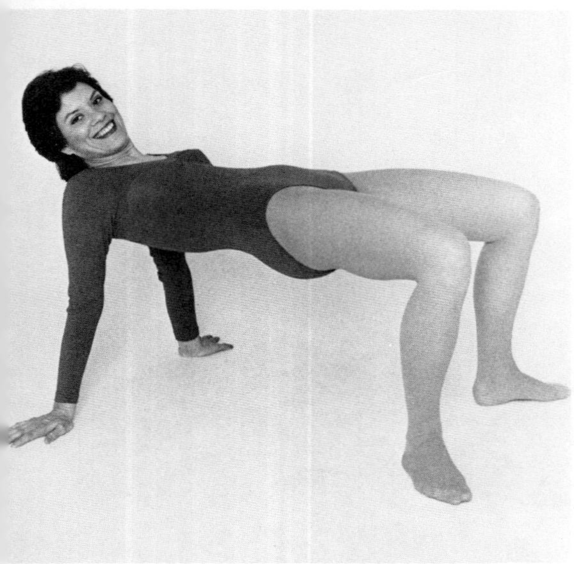

Balance, stomach up, on your hands and feet.

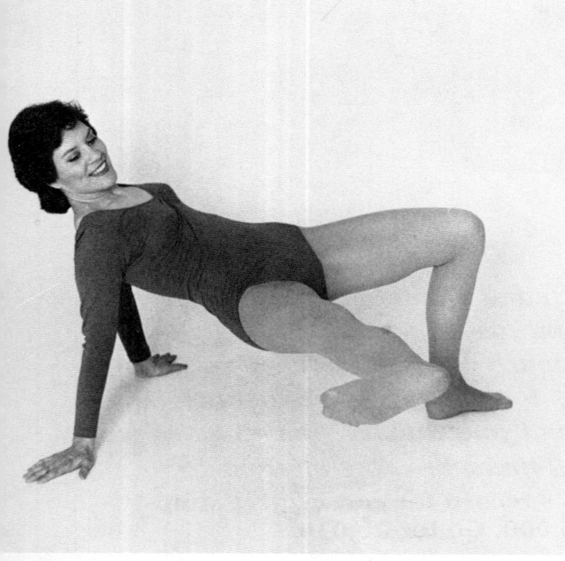

*Now straighten your right leg, lift it until it's level with your stomach, and swing it outward, parallel to the floor, until it forms a right angle with your other leg. Rotate your outstretched leg until the inner thigh faces the ceiling and flex that foot hard. This is the **START** position.*

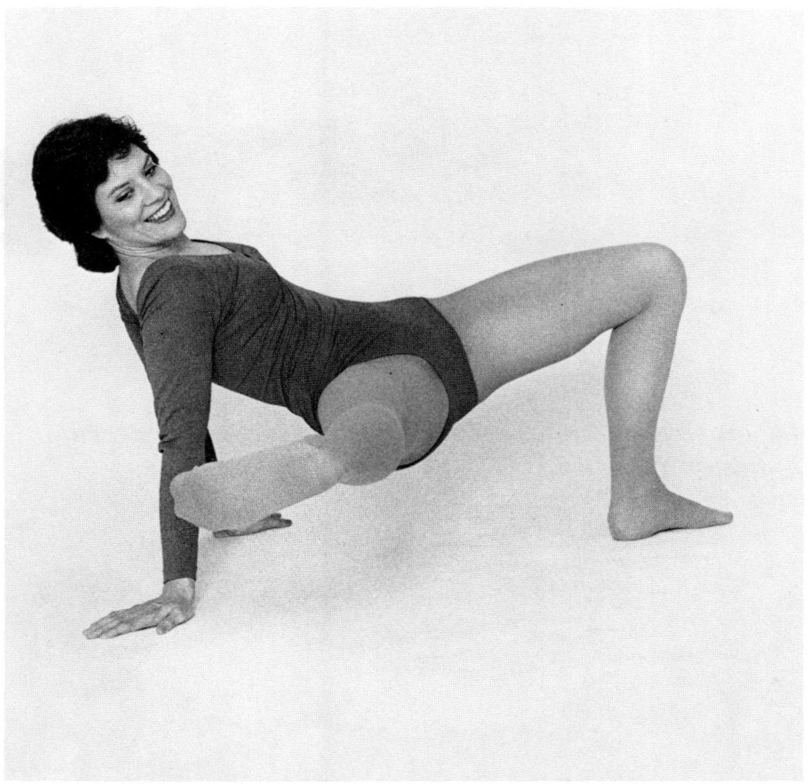

*Now **PUSH** your foot toward your shoulder briskly and as hard as you can 30 times. Repeat 30 times with left leg extended. Feel inner thighs ache-and-shake? Terrific. You hit the spot.*

Helpful hint: If you can't lift your body immediately to start, keep your rear on the floor for the first few days. When you're lifted, you'll notice a bonus ache on the top of the supporting thigh. Fun!

7 The Rump-Raiser Rock

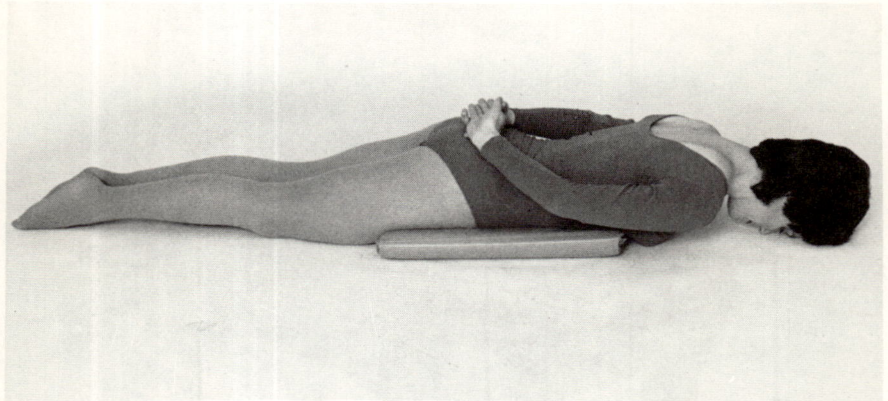

Lie on your cushion on your stomach, legs outstretched, hands on rear. ***READY.***

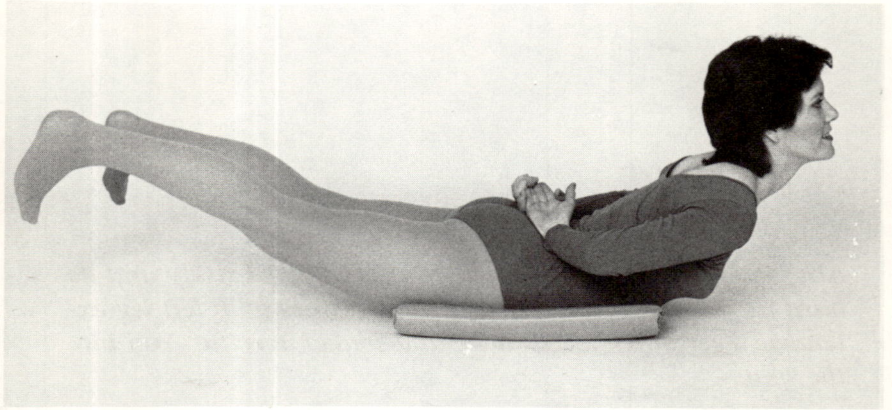

Flex feet hard. Lift arms, legs, thighs, shoulders and upper torso off the floor and ***HOLD THAT ARCH****. This is the* ***START*** *position.*

Helpful hint: If you need some momentum to get started, push your torso up with your hands.

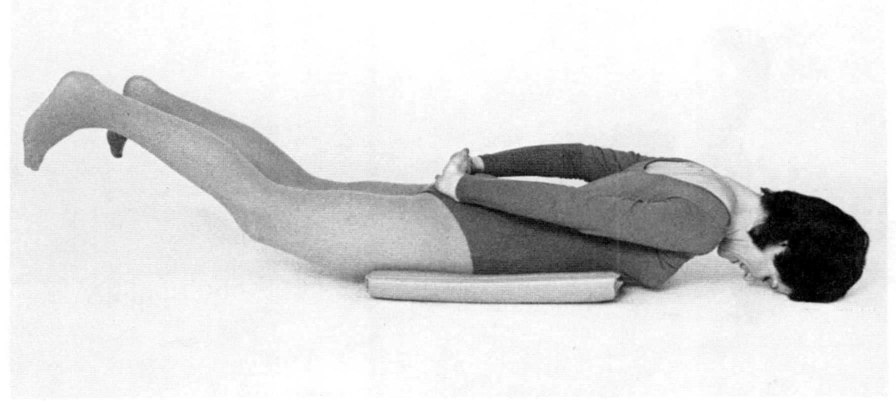

Rock forward until your head touches the floor and. . .

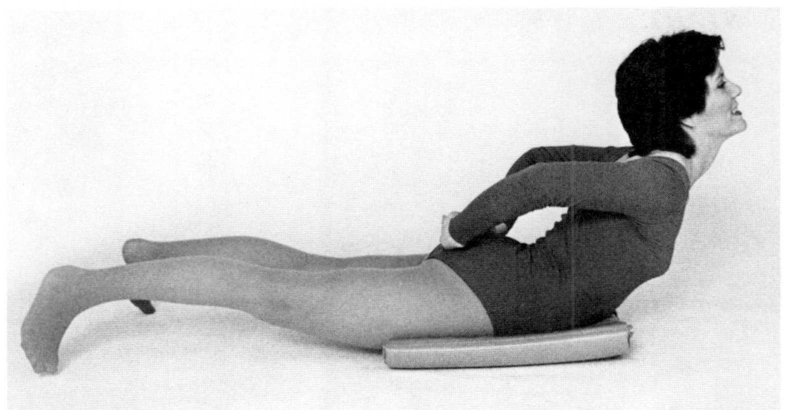

backward until your toes touch the floor. Rock rapidly forward and backward 30 times. Feel derriere sizzle? Right on target!

Note: **There is no known world's record for consecutive rump-raiser rocks. Set one.**

8 *Pushups (New! For Women!)*

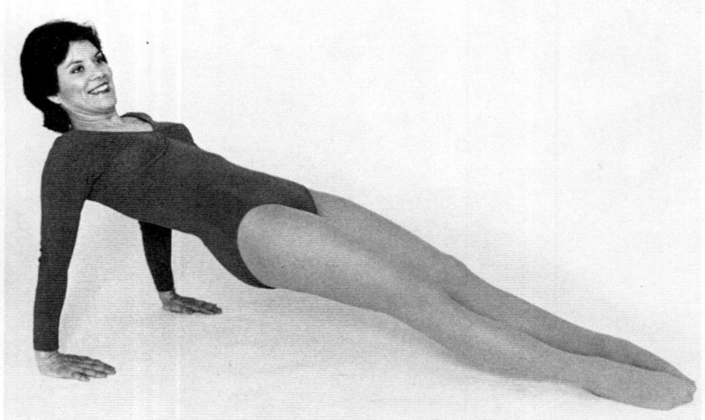

Form a slantboard with your body, balanced on your hands and heels, nose pointed at the ceiling, fingertips pointed toward toes. This is START.

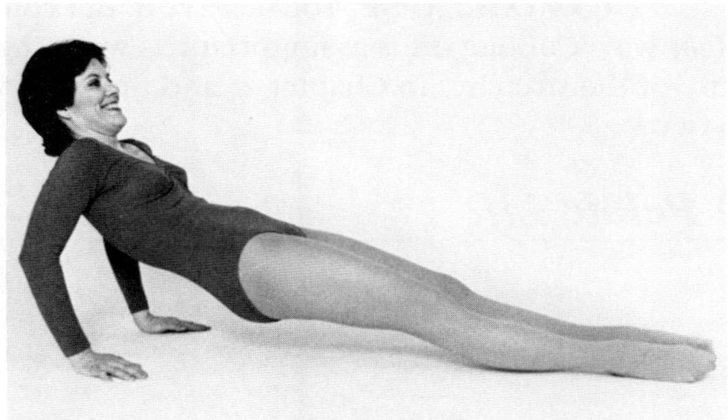

Keeping your body in a straight line, ***BEND YOUR ELBOWS*** *about 4 inches. Straighten them and repeat 20 times. Rejoice as the ache-and-shake shrinks the hanging gardens of the upper arm! Note:* **World's record nonstop pushups: 9,105. Go for it.**

*N*ow **COLLAPSE**. You deserve it. But collapse the *right* way. Cooling off is as important as warming up. Use any of the stretches in Chapter 4, and finish up with these two:

The Pelvic Lift

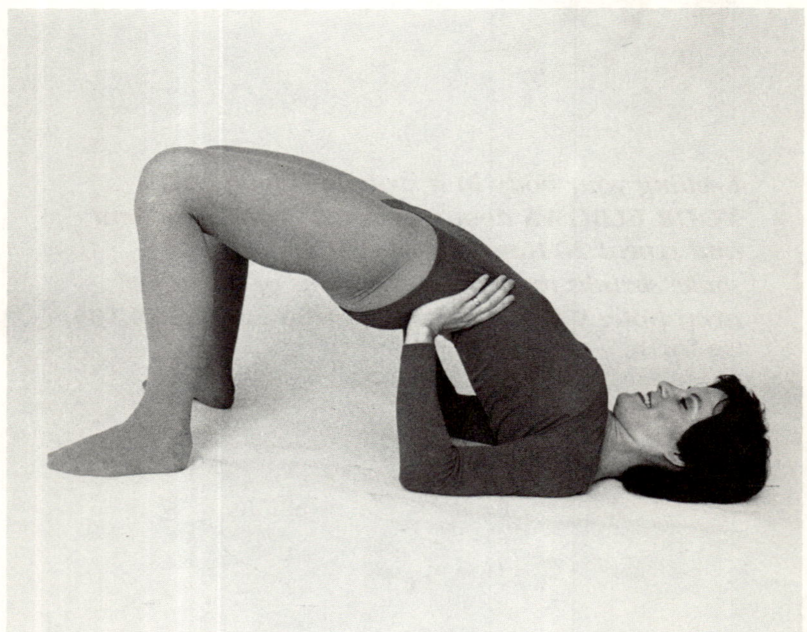

A soothing stretch for your stomach as well as your spine. Lie on your back with knees bent, and slowly roll your pelvis up off the floor until you're supported by your shoulders. Put your hands beneath your waist and gently push your back higher. Lower your back to the floor and pull yourself into:

The All-Purpose Curl

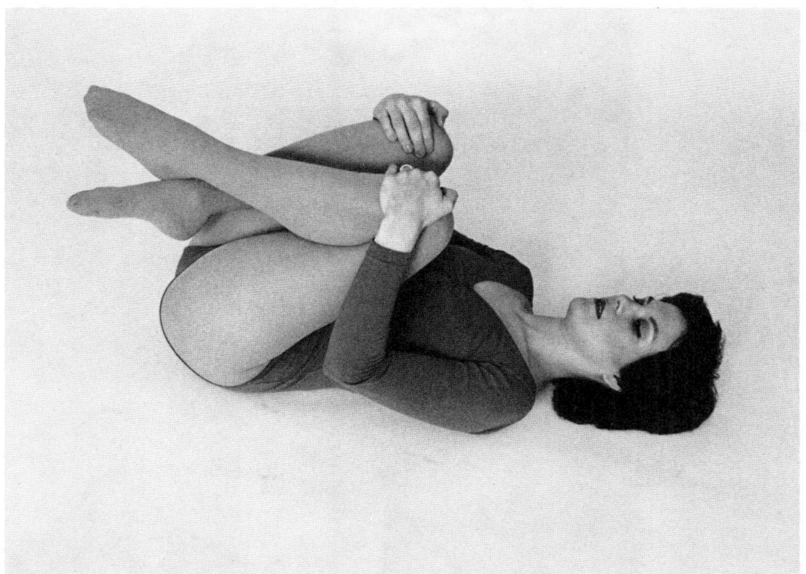

A lovely little do-it-yourself back massage (which you can use at any time during your routine). Lie flat with your back and head on the floor. Grab your knees and gently pull them toward your chest. Pull, relax. Pull, relax. A-a-a-h-h-h.

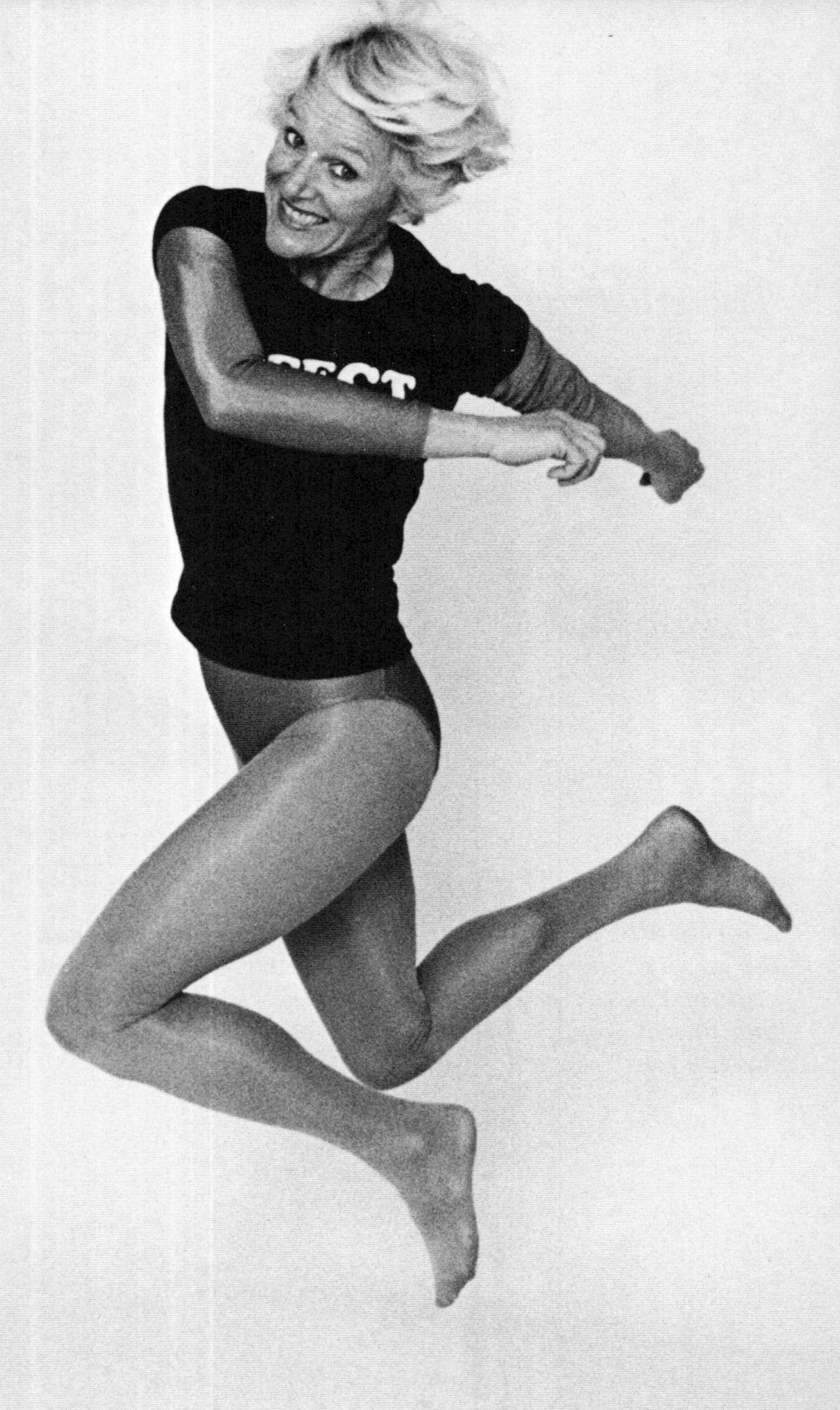

3 *Moving to Perfection*

You did it!

Just three weeks have passed, and you can wear a smaller skirt, a smaller shirt, and you can zip up last year's jeans without breaking all your fingernails.

What next? Perfection, of course! A skimpy swimsuit.

You are now ready to shed the remaining mush, to create an even leaner you—to move into your perfect body.

You are ready to be a Prime Mover.

The Prime Move System is slightly different.

You give yourself 4–5 weeks more, you make your Moves only four times a week, you use only four Moves—variations of the Basic 8.

1 The Bigger Big Leap

*E*xpand your leap to 35 minutes, nonstop. Five minutes of jog warmup, 27 minutes in second and high gear, 3 minutes geardown. Now you can *fly*!

Tour Jeté

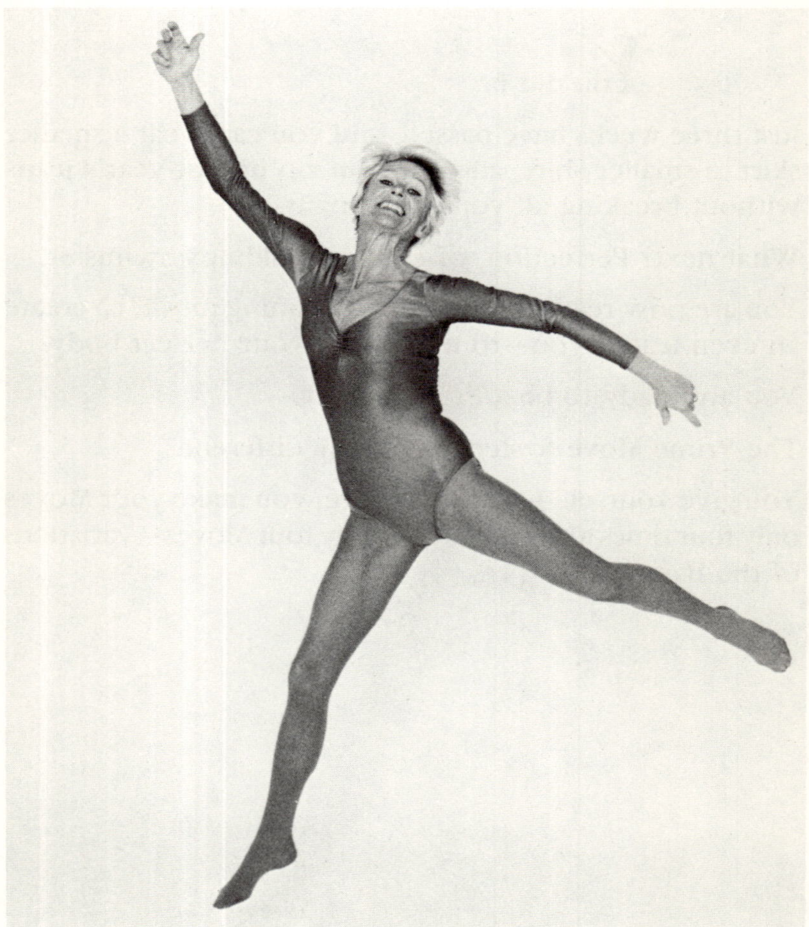

Use all your original leaps and add 10 minutes of these: be a star! Make a few tour jeté ***entrances, feed in some . . .***

Entrechat

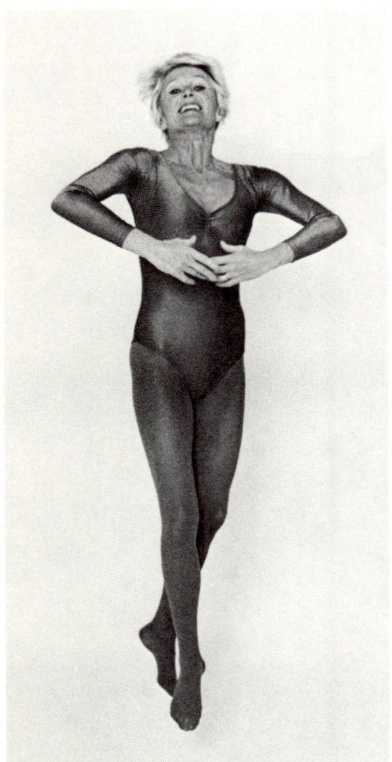

***entrechats**, then click your heels together in mid-air and shout:*

Oklahoma Heel Click

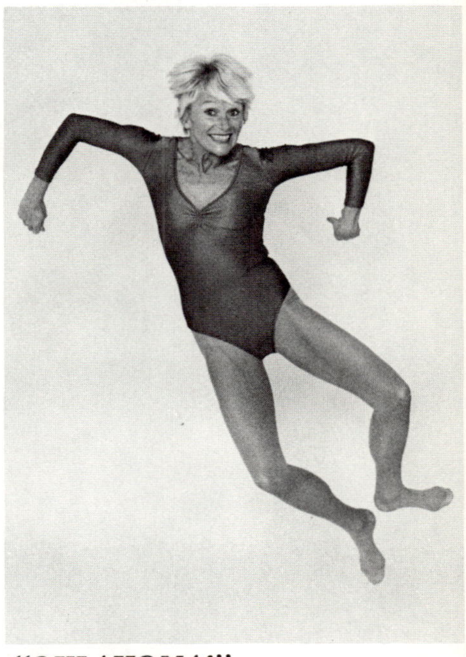

"OKLAHOMA!"

Cakewalk

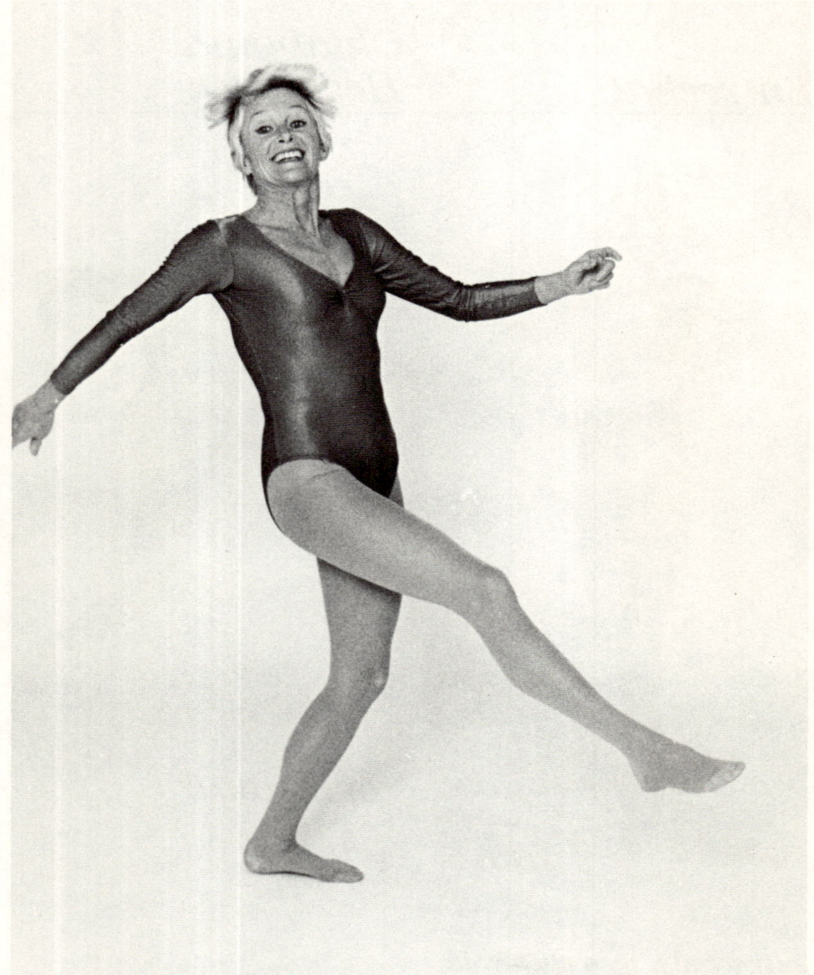

Don't just strut down Bourbon Street. ***Cakewalk*** *up Fifth Avenue!*

Highland Fling | *Flamenco*

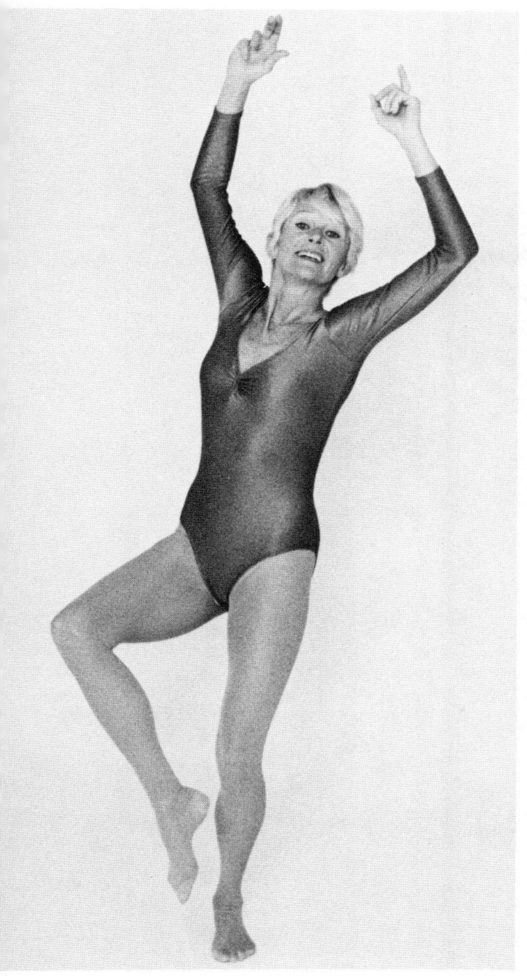

*Move around the world: do the **Highland Fling**. . . .*

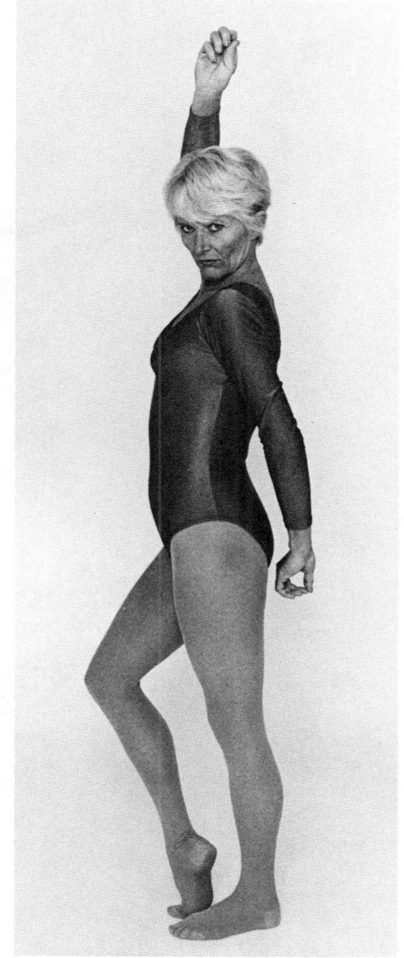

*the **Flamenco**. . .*

Limbo

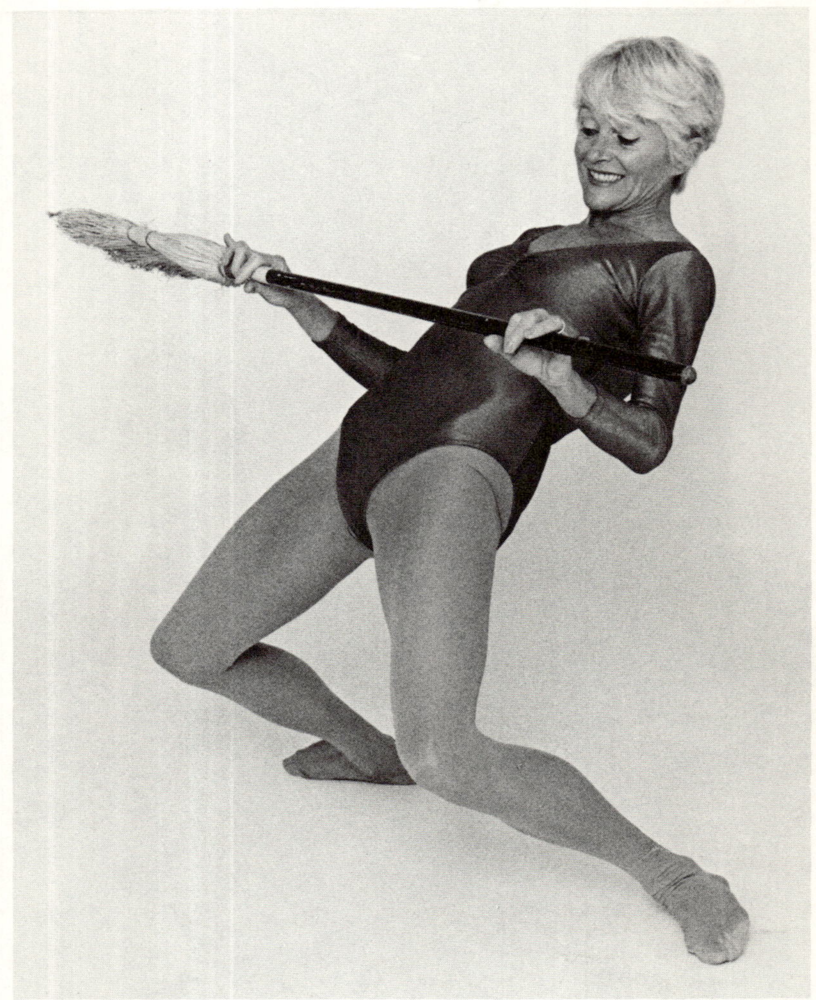

the Limbo!

Leapfrog

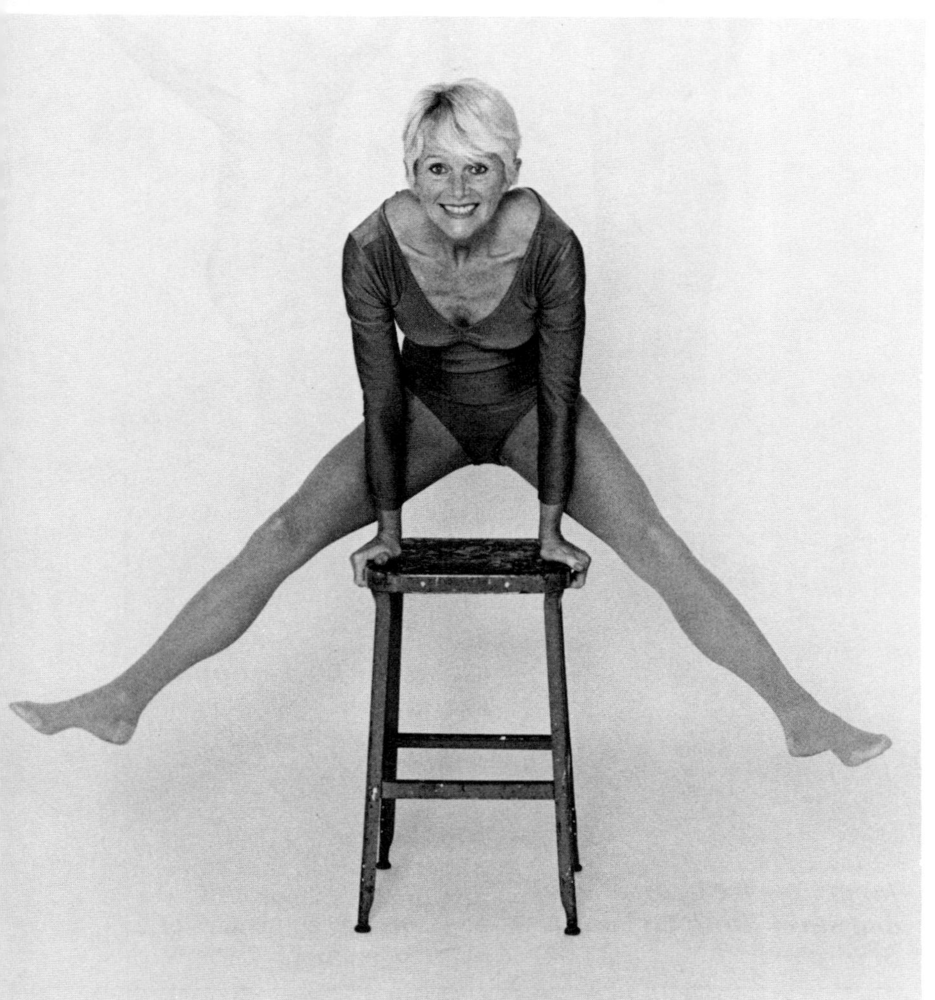

Play games: ***Leapfrog*** *over the furniture . . .*

Slam Dunk

Punt

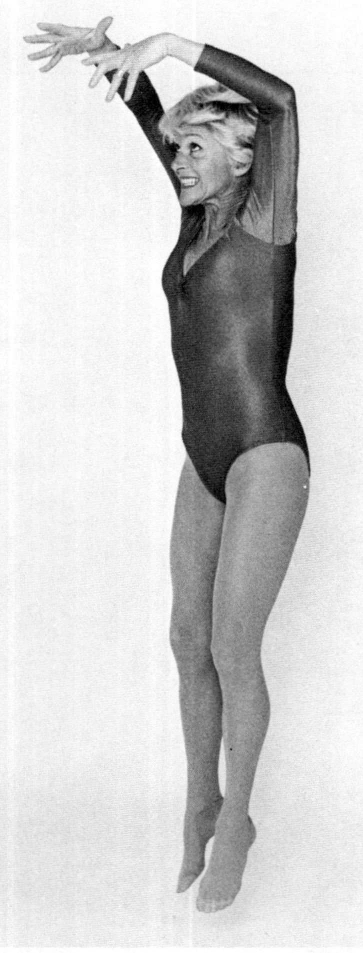

jump over the guards' heads and ***slam dunk*** *50 baskets in a row. . .*

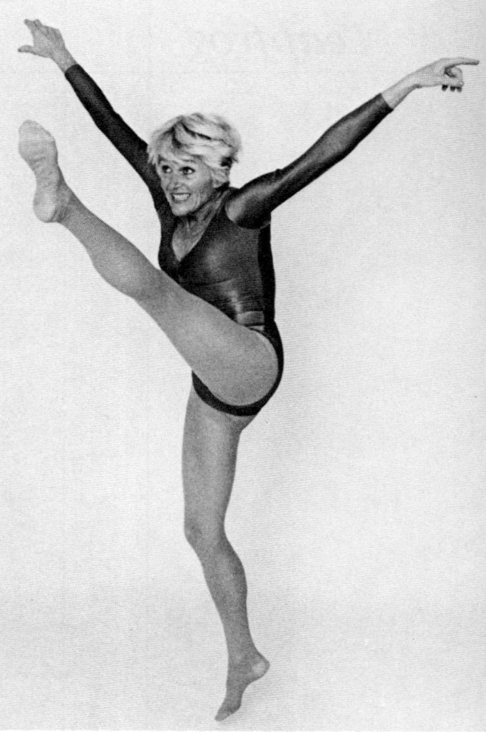

Kick a few 99-yard ***punts! Run amok!***

Alternatives to this Move: a *very brisk* 1½-hour walk, a 3-mile jog, or 20 minutes of nonstop jumprope.

Note: **The world's fastest flamenco dancer pounded out 1,000 heel taps per minute. Pound faster! The world's record for continuous high kicks is 8,491—kick more and higher! The world's longest punt, 98 yards, was made by Steve O'Neal of the New York Jets in 1969. Kick him out of the record book!**

2 *The Balanced Paunch-Puncher Pullup with Leg Action*

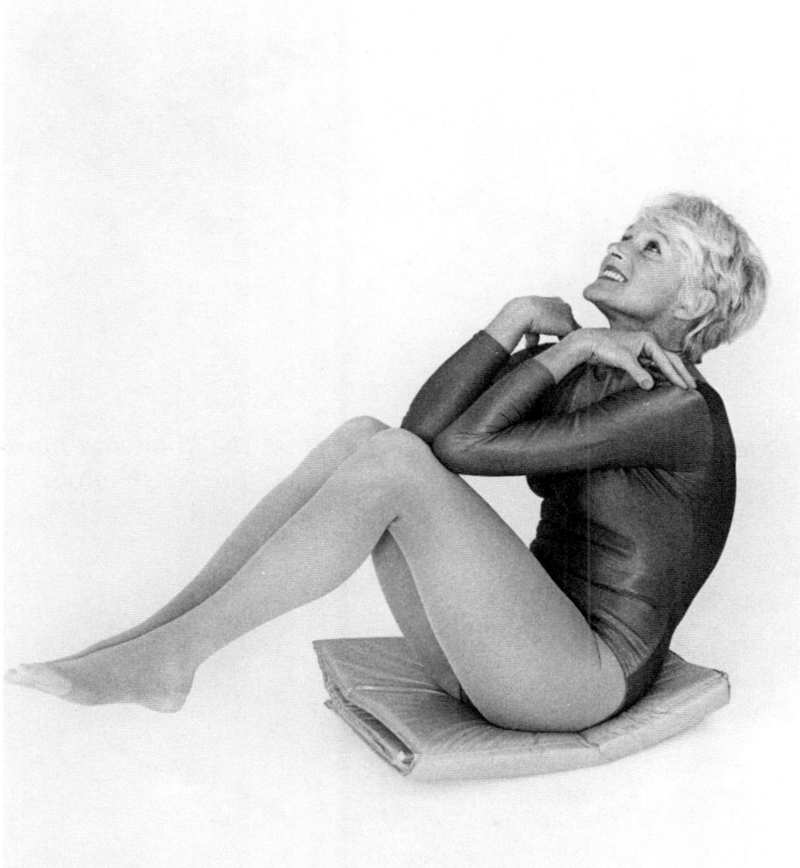

Balance on your rear, fingertips on shoulders, knees touching elbows.

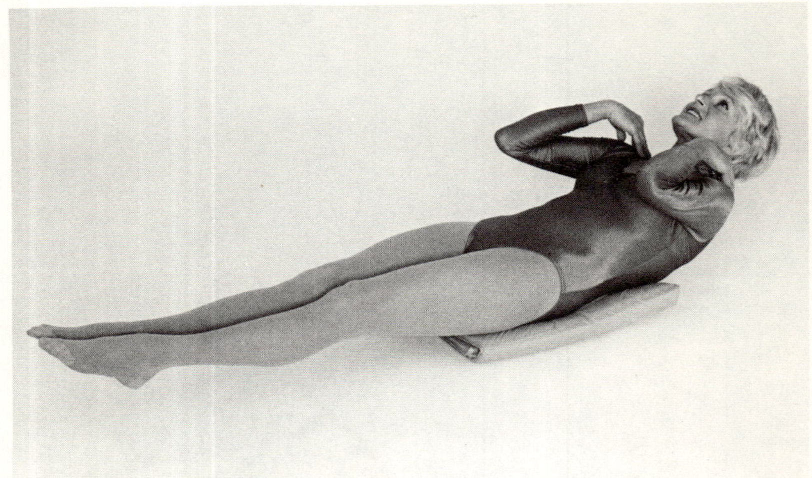

Extend your legs to about 6 inches from the floor and lower your trunk until the small of your back touches the floor.

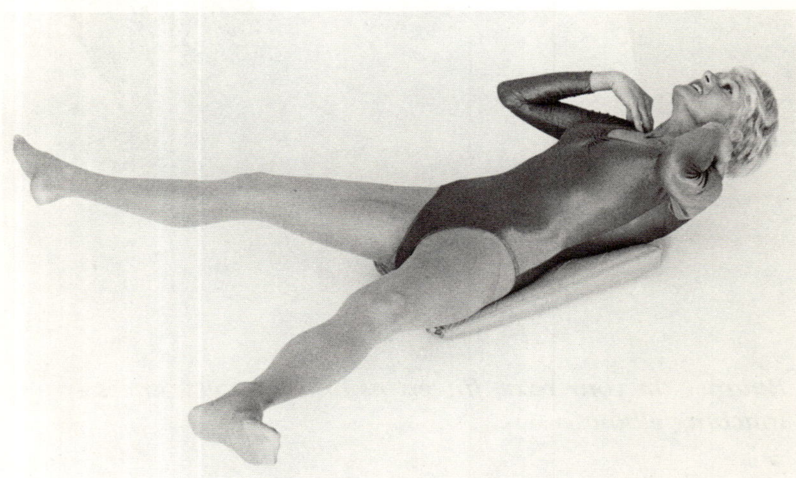

***Now ADD THE LEG ACTION:** turn your toes out, separate your legs as wide as you can, then. . .*

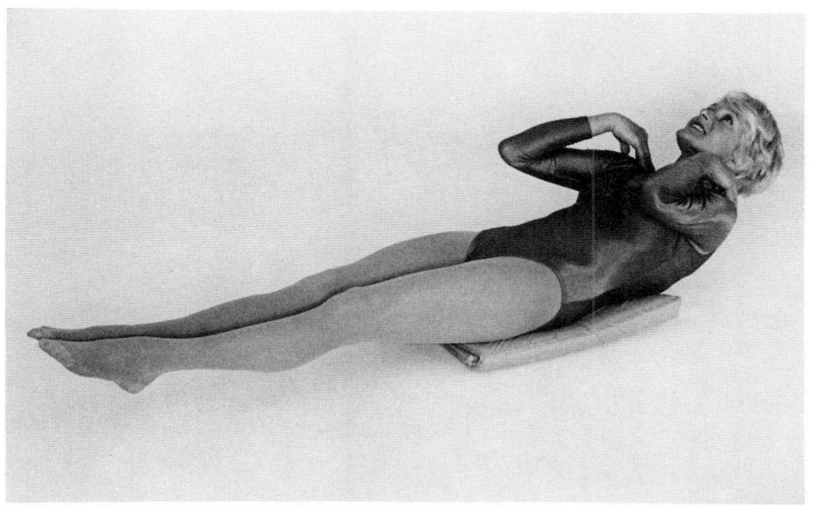

bring them together again.

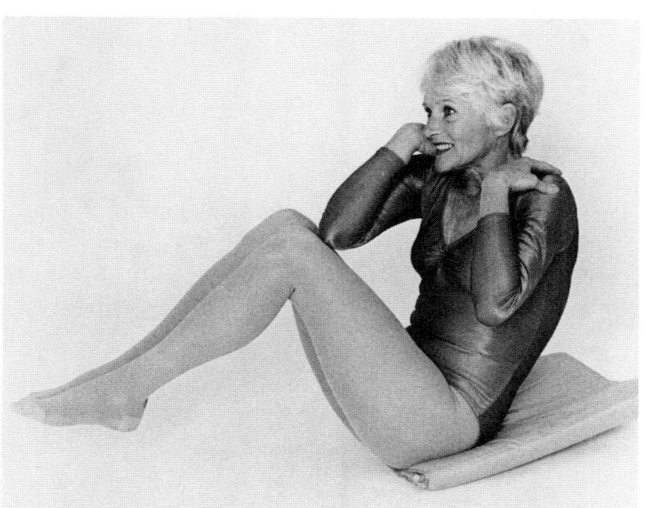

Pull legs and trunk up, twist and touch right elbow to left knee. Build to 30 repetitions, alternating elbow to opposite knee.

*Wasn't the basic paunch-puncher **boring?***

3 The Stretched-Out Rump-Raiser Rock

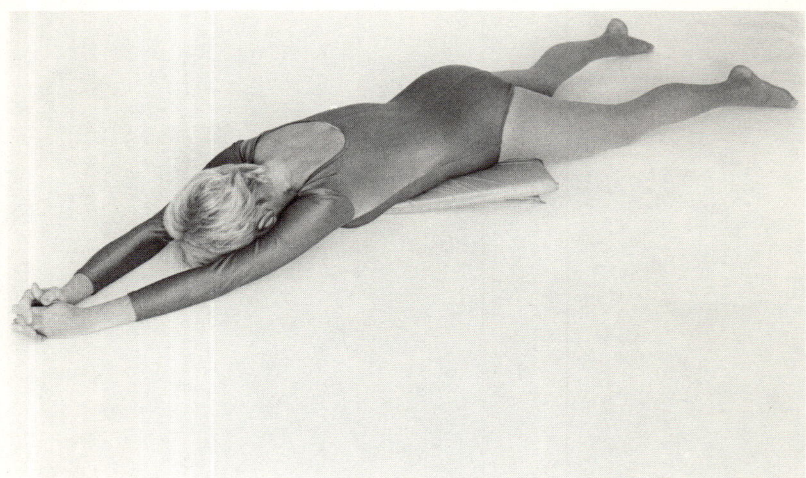

Lie on your cushion on your stomach, arms and legs outstretched and straight.

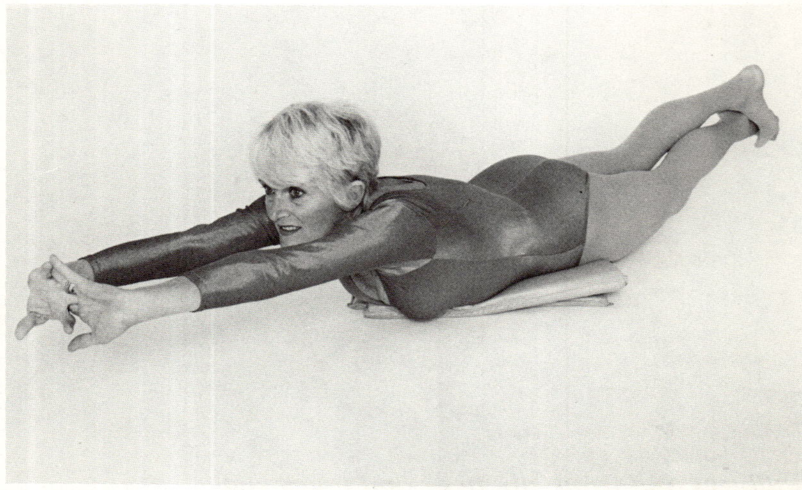

Cross feet. Lift arms, legs, thighs, shoulders and upper trunk and ***HOLD THAT ARCH****. This is the* ***START*** *position.*

Helpful hint: Make this more interesting. Switch feet positions with *every* rock.

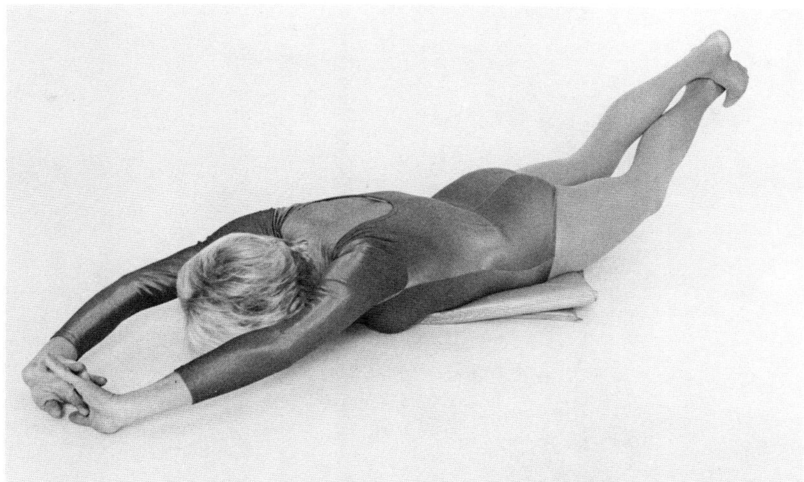

Rock forward until your chin touches the floor and. . .

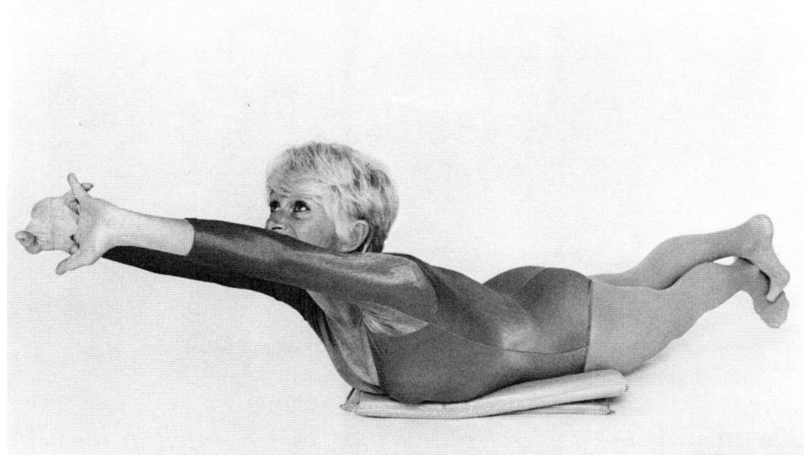

backward until your toes touch the floor. Rock fast, switch feet positions halfway through, and work up from 10 to 30 repetitions.

4 The Legs-Up Diaphragm-Slam With a Twist and a Clap

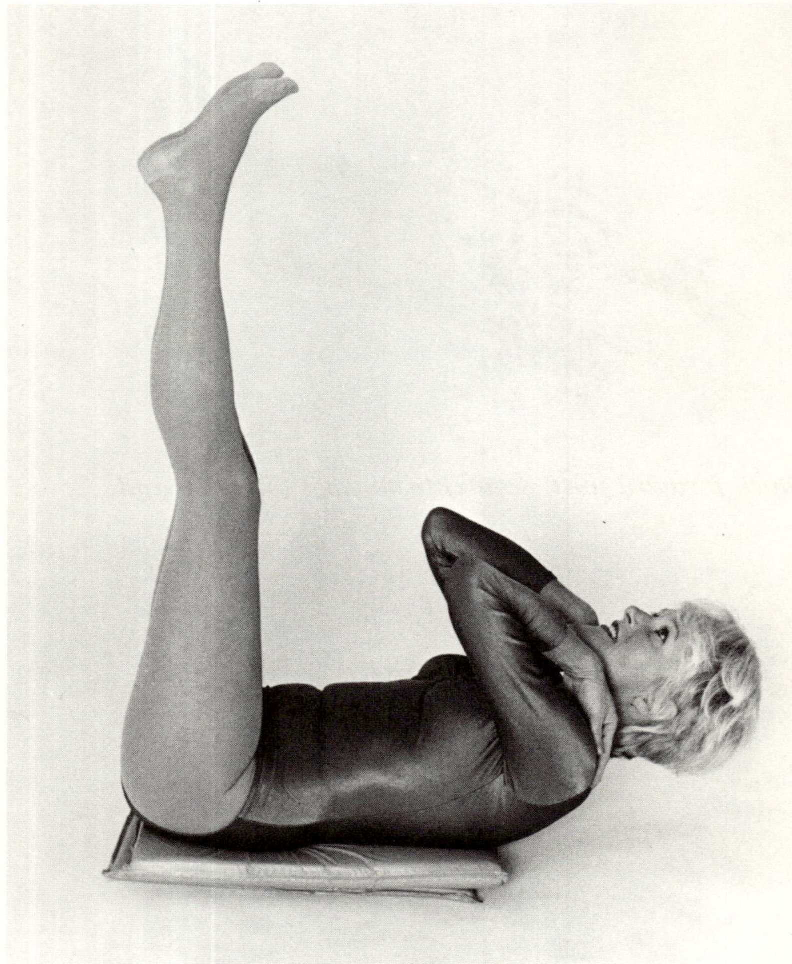

Lie on your back with legs together, toes pointed at the ceiling, fingertips on shoulders and elbows pointed at knees.

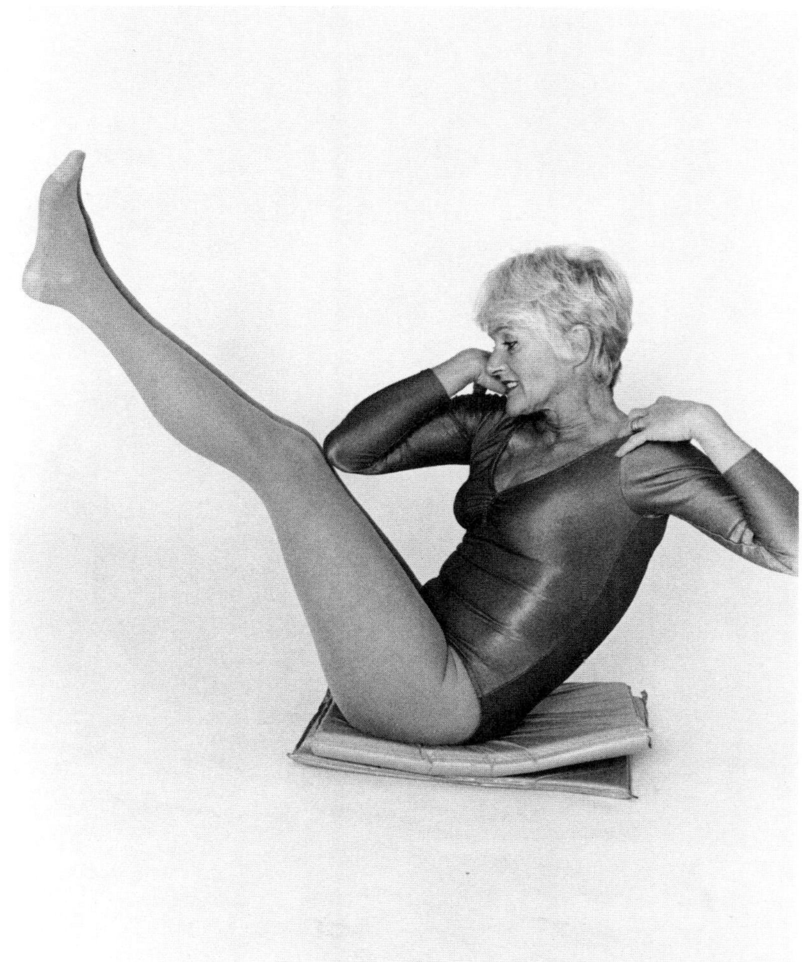

Lift your torso until your right elbow touches your left knee.

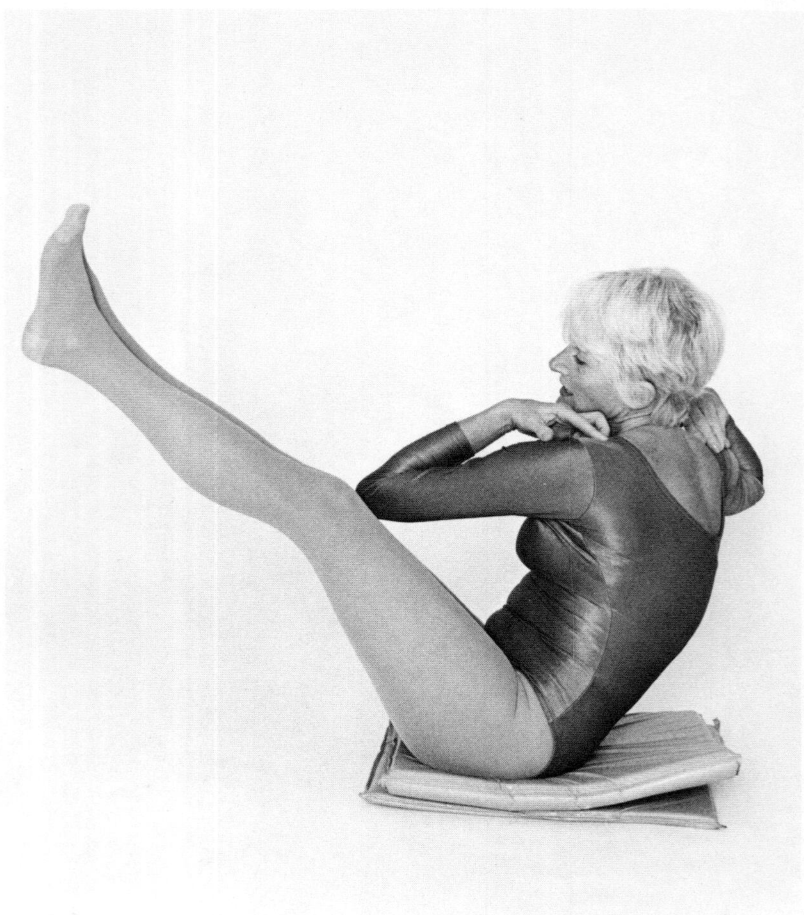

Hold the lift and touch left elbow to right knee.

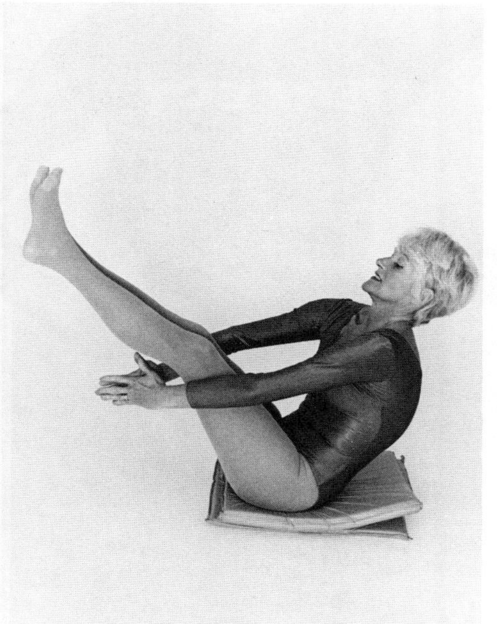

Still holding, clap your hands behind your legs.

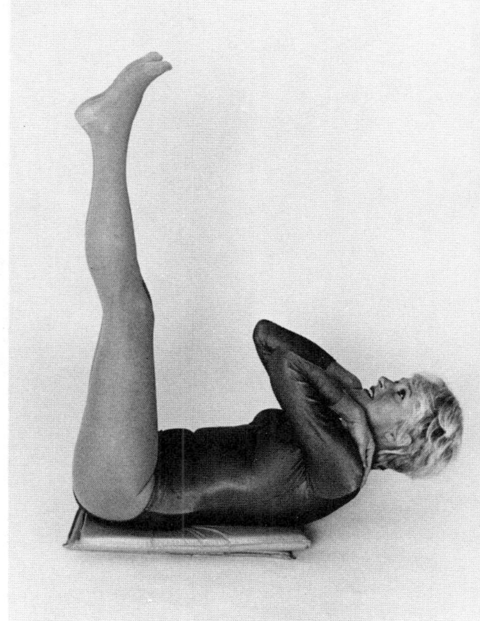

Lower your back (but not your head) to the mat. Work up to 30 fast repetitions.

Note: **The world's record for longest continuous clapping—140 claps per minute audible at 100 yards—is 42 hours, 6 minutes. Consider throwing this in for variety.**

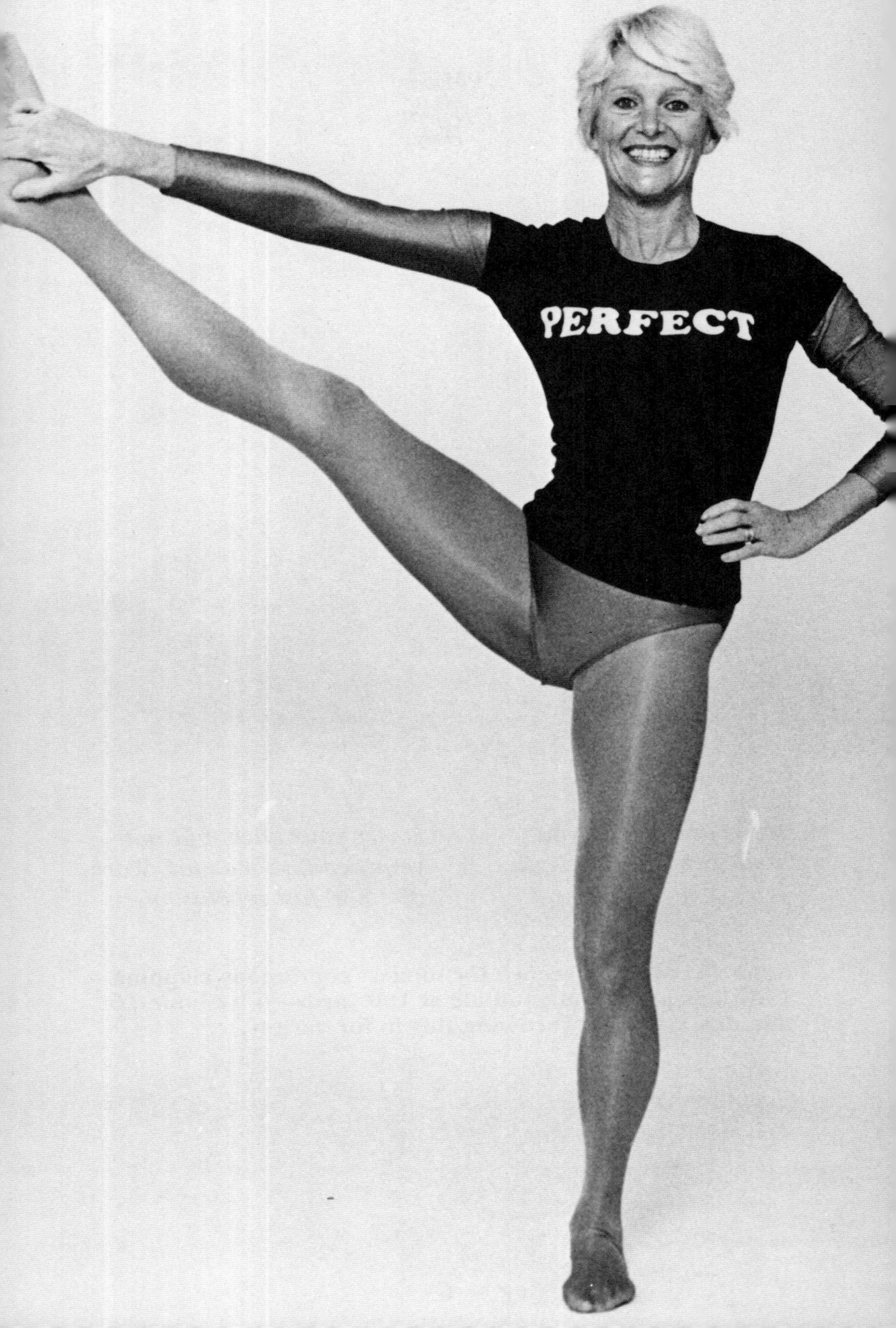

PERFECT

4 Moving Loose and Moving Wisely

Whether you're moving with the Basic 8 or the 4 Prime Moves, your perfect body needs one more ingredient: flexibility.

Never mind that you can now lift your own weight 20 times over, like a tiny brave ant carrying a giant mantis to its burrow. Can you touch your toes without crying?

(Well, can you?)

Flexibility means being loose in the connective tissue around your bone joints, including muscles, tendons and ligaments.

The elasticity and the length of these tissues mean the difference between good, natural movement—or clumsiness, stiffness, and *hurt*.

Most infamous problem areas: lower back, shoulders, hamstrings (backs of legs) and Achilles tendons (backs of ankles).

You don't have to be a contortionist to be flexible, but you can have fun with it.

Try my four favorite stretches. Do them *SLOWLY*, and hold for only 5–10 seconds at a *slight discomfort* (not a *screaming*) point. I don't have to tell you what they stretch—you'll know when you try them.

1 My Favorite Stretches

The Deferential Stork

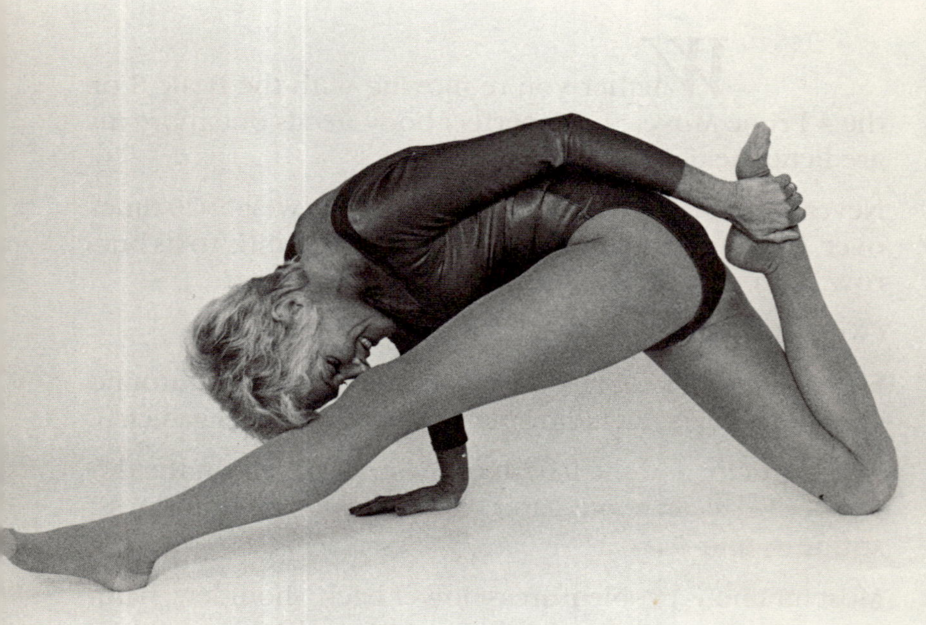

The Timid Turkey

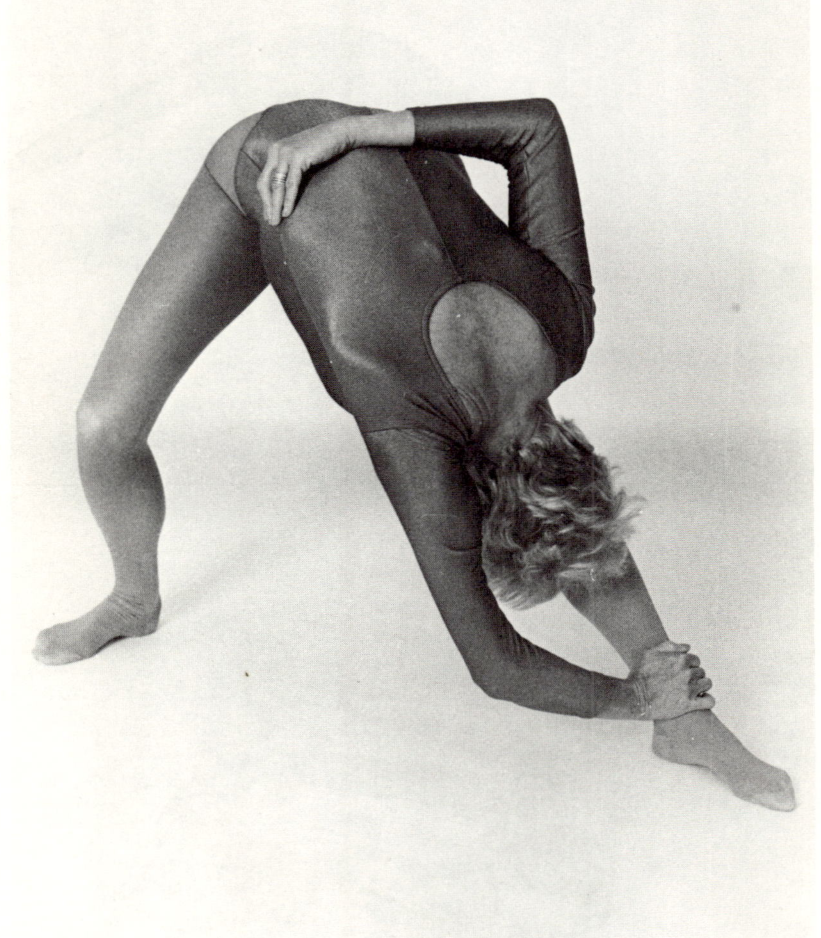

The Gibbon

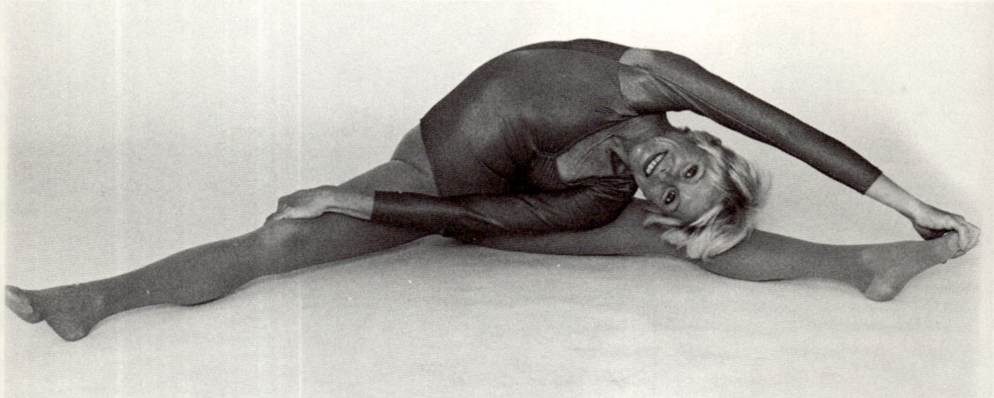

The Flying Frog

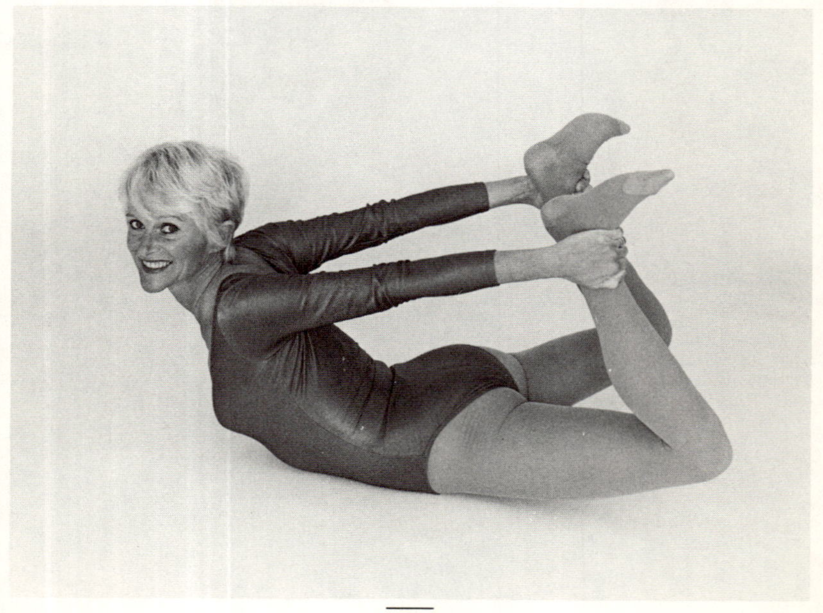

2 Exercise No-Nos:

Being loose is one way to avoid hurting your perfect body. Another is to avoid certain specific exercises.

No Duck Walks or Deep Knee Bends

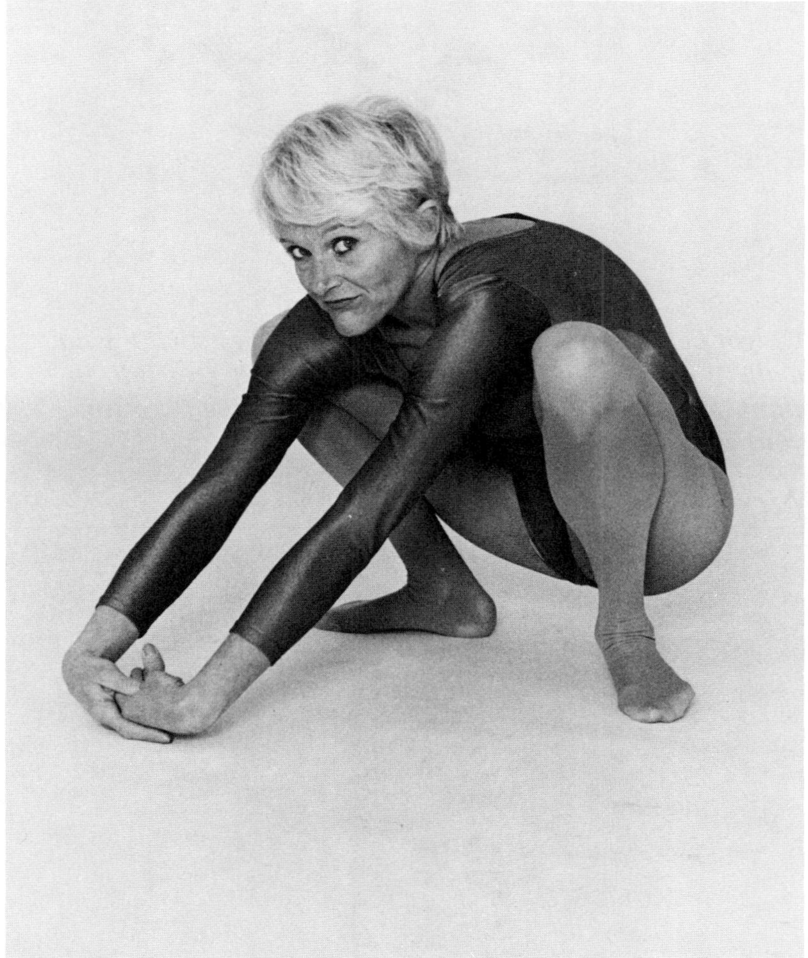

This was the first exercise to be condemned by the President's Council on Physical Fitness. Quack your way to torn knee cartilage.

No Gimmicky Exercise "Aids"

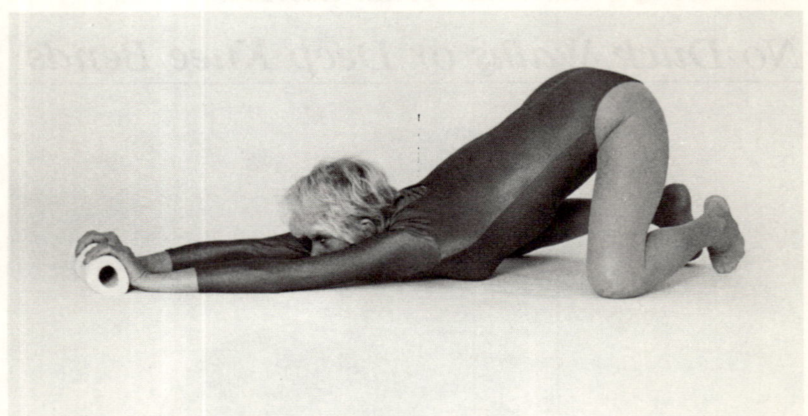

*Weight belts that "melt your fat" (while they shrink your wallet); rubberized workout suits (that melt **you** into instant dehydration); things you push along the floor (on your way to orthopedic surgery).*

No Hurdler's Stretch

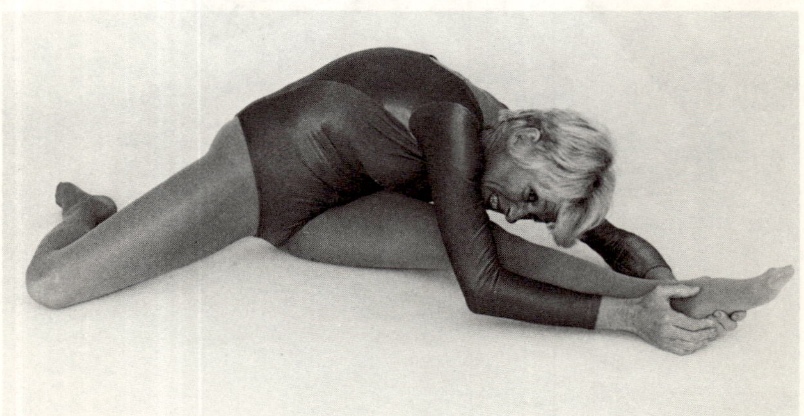

Two million runners can be wrong. This one can wreak havoc on your knees, flog sciatic nerves, and cause chronic groin pull. Ouch!

No Facial "Exercises"

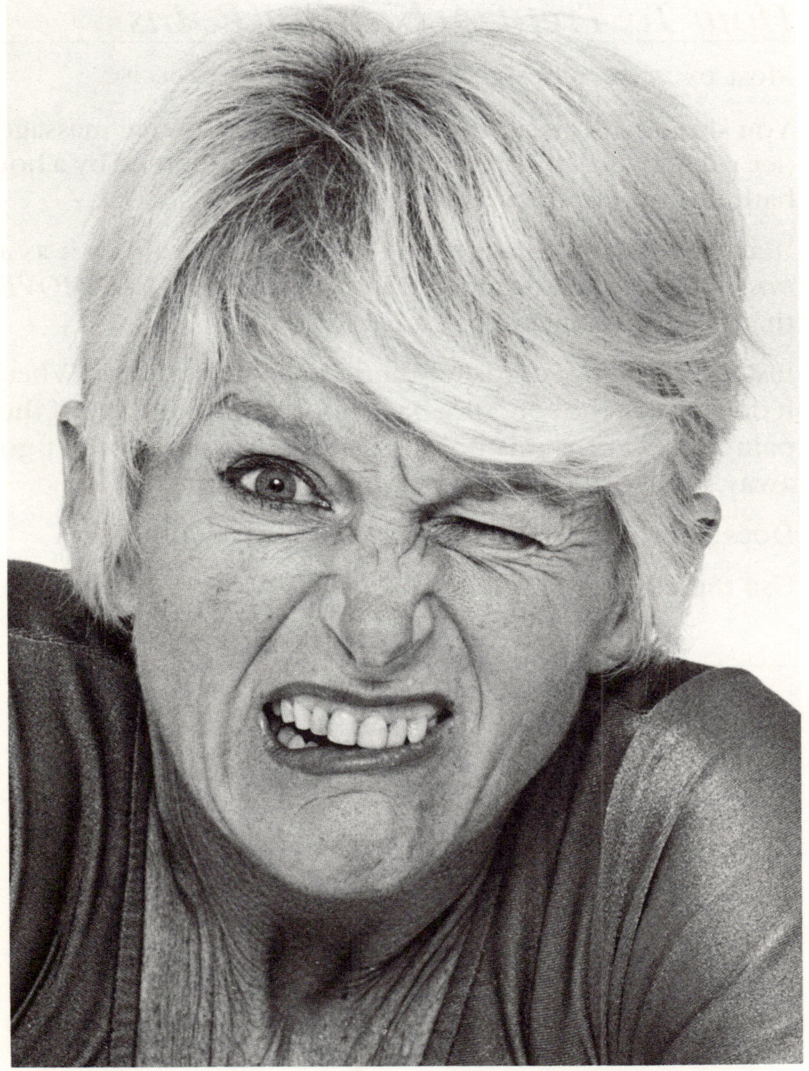

Gravity does enough to your face without any help from you. Keep mugging, and you'll be checking in for a lift long before you're truly due.

How To Treat Aches and Pains

Most exercise aches go away with more exercise.

You should also treat them with a 10-minute ice massage (ice rubbed directly on the trouble spot), followed by a hot bath and a couple of aspirin before bed.

If an ache becomes a piercing one (which qualifies it as a *pain*), or persists for more than three days, *DON'T MOVE* that part of your body in any exercise.

Just leave it alone completely until the pain goes away. When it does, work the sore spot back into shape gradually. If the pain reappears at this point, is still sharp, and doesn't go away immediately, check with your doctor.

Does your perfect back ache from time to time?

Use these Spine Soothers and pat it!

3 *Pats for Aching Backs*

The Cat

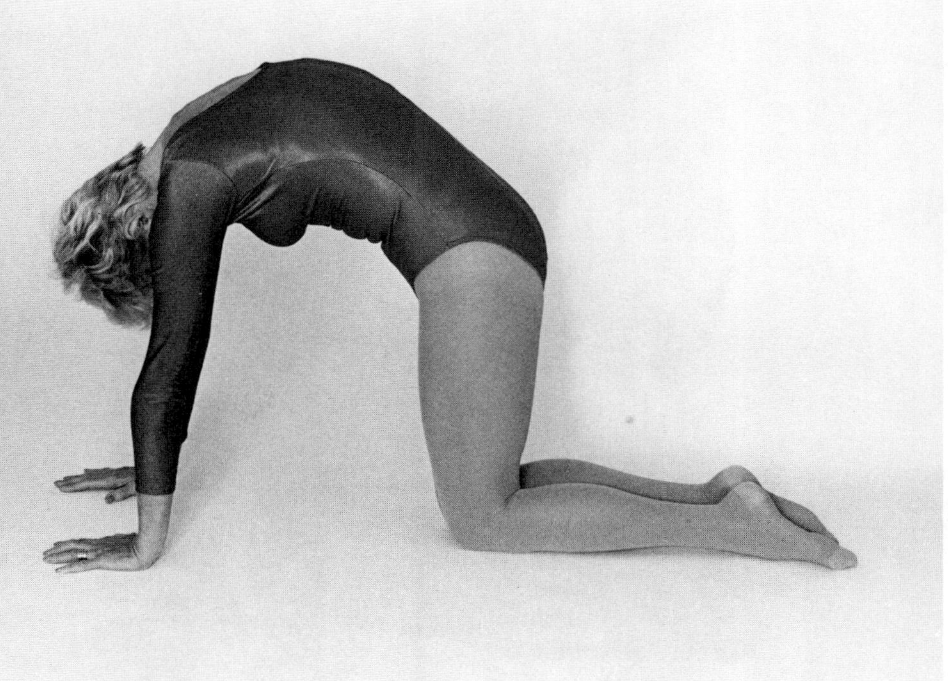

*Push your back **SLOWLY** up into a Halloween cat hump, suck in your stomach, let your head hang heavily, breathe easily and hold for 10 seconds. Alternate upward pushes with slow sags into a swayback.*

The Bat

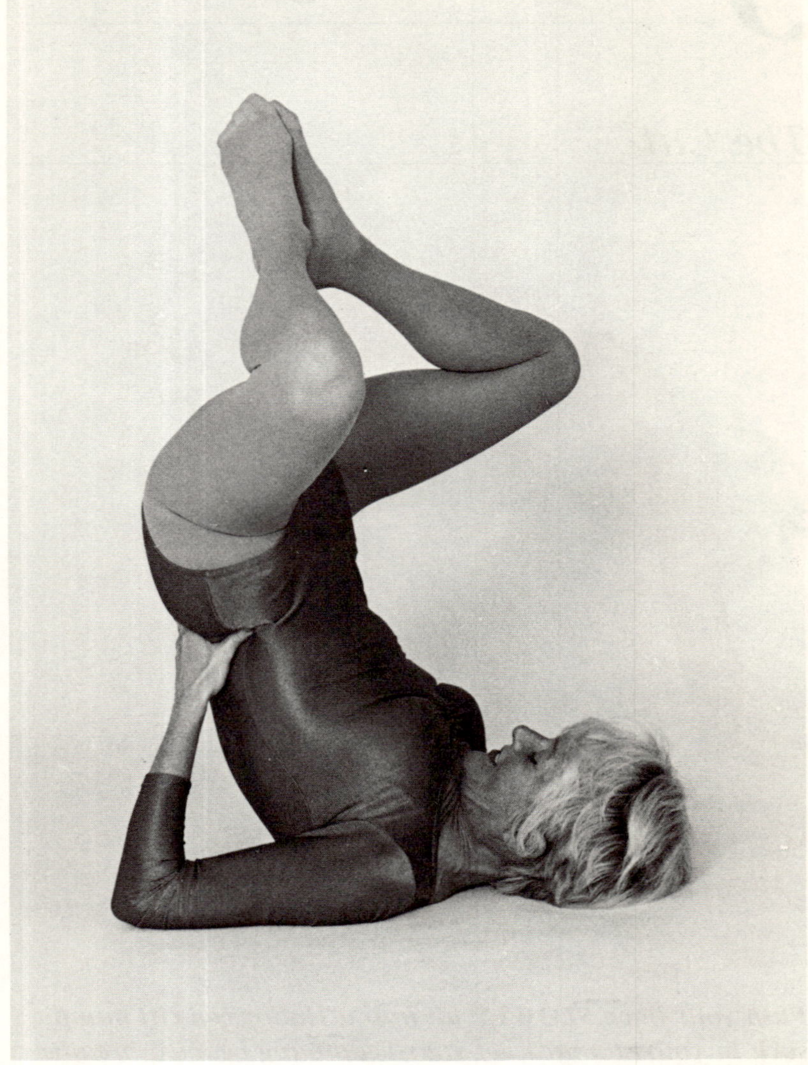

A sloppy Yoga shoulder stand. Roll up onto your shoulders, supporting your back with your hands, and let your knees dangle over your nose in a comfort zone. Don't put any weight onto your neck or head. If you're bored, count the rolls on your stomach.

The Lazy Ostrich

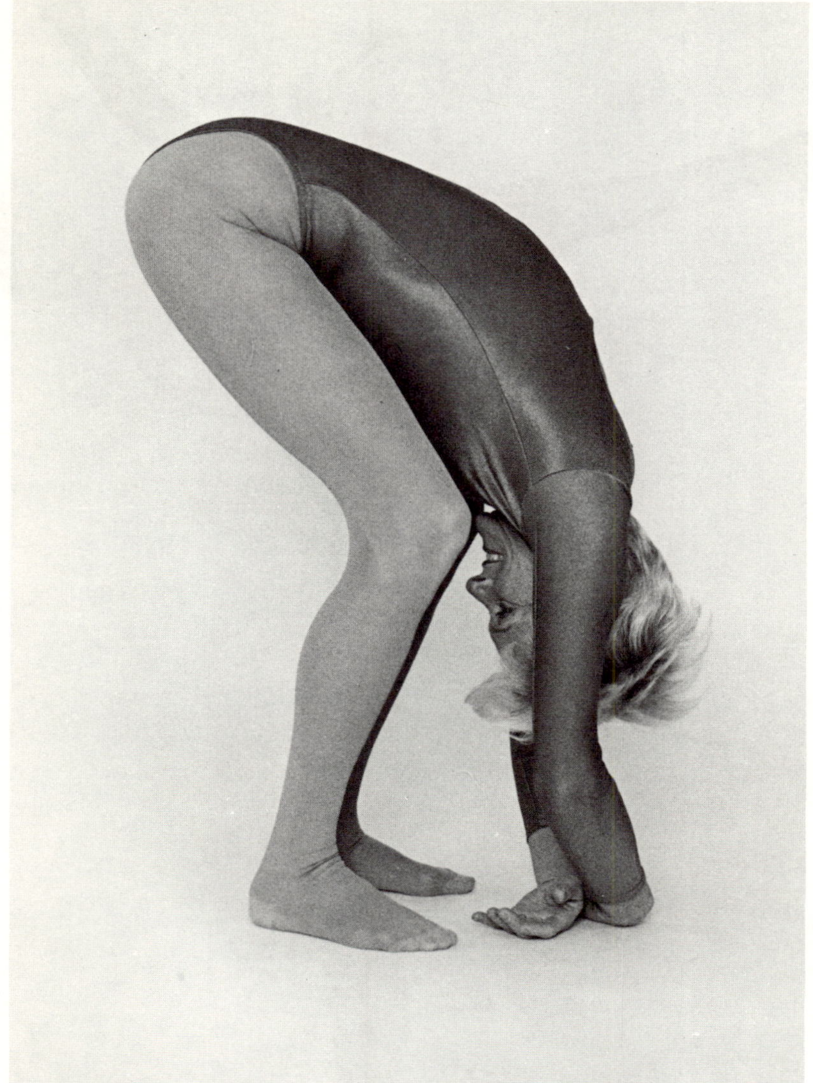

Stand. Bend your knees and slowly bend forward, keeping your head, shoulders, and hands ***very*** *heavy. Your head weighs 12–15 pounds. Use it to stretch out that spine. Hang. Delicious.*

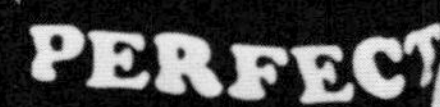
PERFECT

5 Moving Ahead

Moving ahead means **KEEP MOVING**.

For good. For the rest of your life.

Why not? Aren't the rewards delicious?

When you become a regular prime mover, you also drop *years*—from your body, your face, your outlook on life.

You have more staying power, working or playing.

You have an outlet for frustration, a release from anxiety and tension, and a potent weapon against depression.

You know how to beat the everyday blahs or the heavy duty blues: get up and **MOVE**.

Studies have shown that this mood-elevating side effect of vigorous exercise may have a physiological basis.

There are substances in our brains called "endorphins," which have a chemical structure similar to morphine—and, like opiates, can kill pain or cause feelings of euphoria.

The studies showed that endorphin levels rise sharply after hard exercise. The implication: the more you move, the greater your output of "natural pleasure chemicals."

Exercise is a weapon against a host of diseases. It reduces chances of strokes or heart attacks; it may hold off other forms of heart disease, such as atherosclerosis; it is recommended for diabetes control. It reduces varicose veins.

It helps regulate menstrual, menopausal, and sleep disorders.

And (whoopee!) exercise limits the physical deterioration of aging.

The average sedentary person gains a pound of body weight while losing a half a pound of lean tissue each year from age 35 to 65. But, since exercise builds lean tissue, regular workouts slow or even stop this process.

Older people who work out regularly have a "functional age" years below their chronological age.

Consider Johnny Kelsey, who was 74 in 1982 when he ran his 51st Boston Marathon.

Consider Ruth Goldfarb, at age 81, the oldest woman in recorded sport to ever complete three marathons. (She *started* running at 74.)

Now consider your own navel.

How do you maintain your own perfect body? Easy. Do the Basic 8 Moves, 3–5 times a week. Or more.

The more the merrier.

The more the leaner.

The more you can eat without fear.

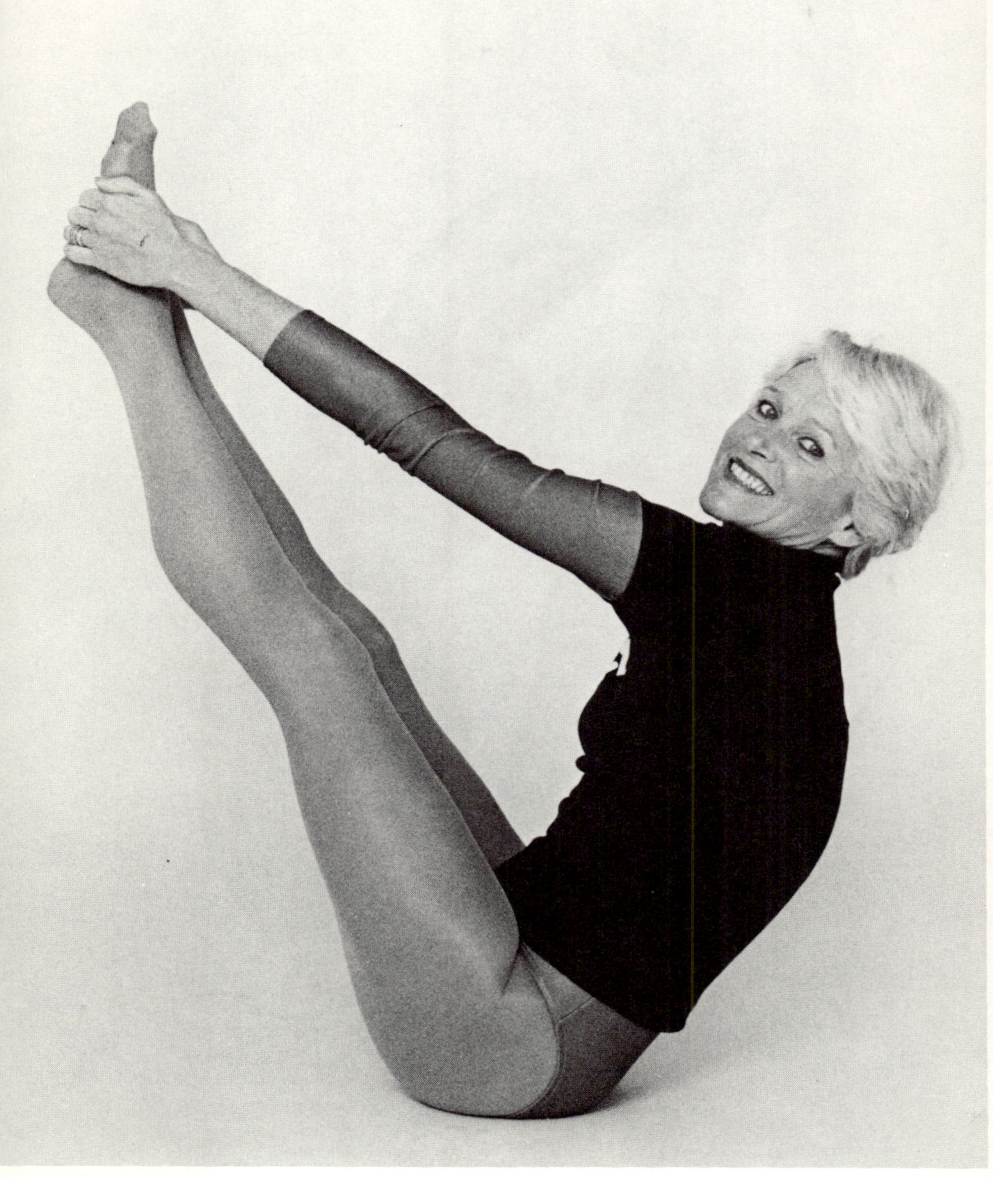

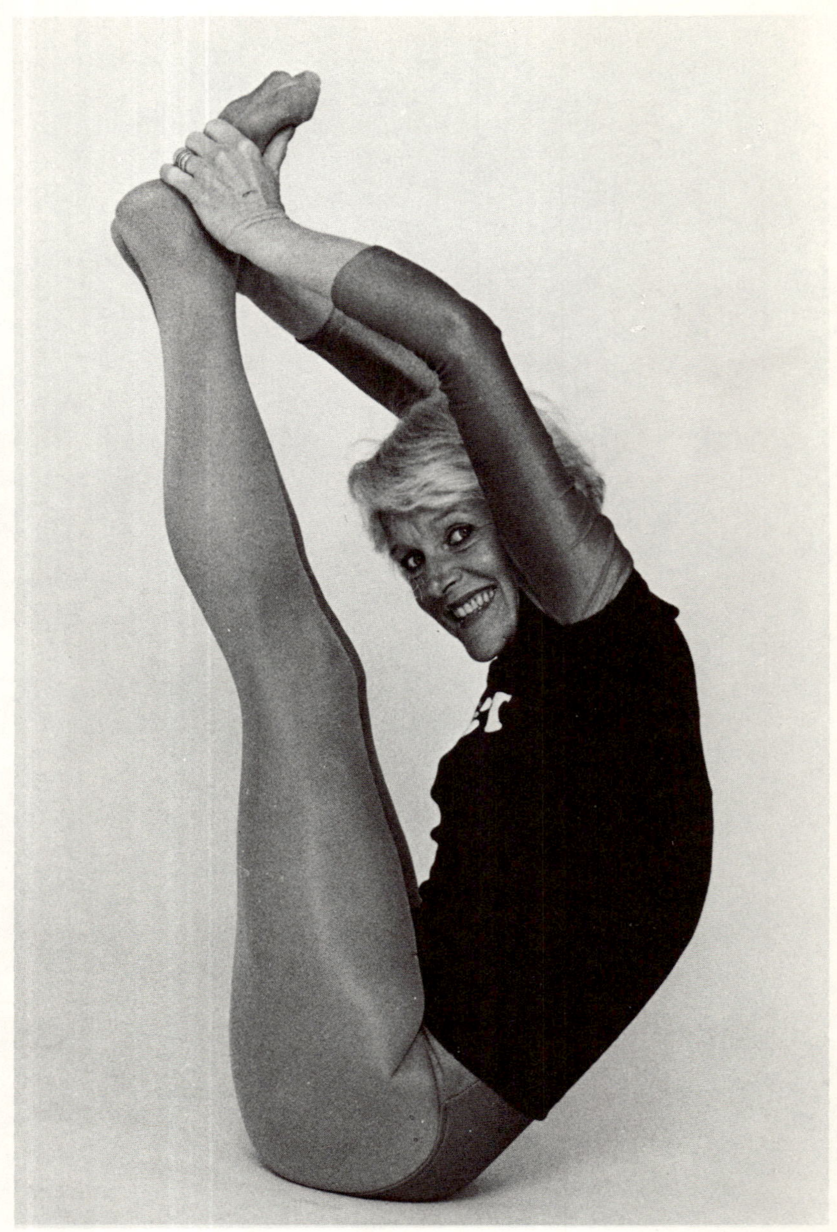

6 The Perfection Plus Pop Quiz

Oh, come on—final exams are *fun*!

Test your perfection level with these Six Bionic Body Builders. (Duck soup after a few weeks with this book.)

There are only two ground rules: first, do them one after the other, *without stopping*; second, keep smiling.

On your mark, get set . . . . follow the photos and go!

1 Two-Hand Body Lift

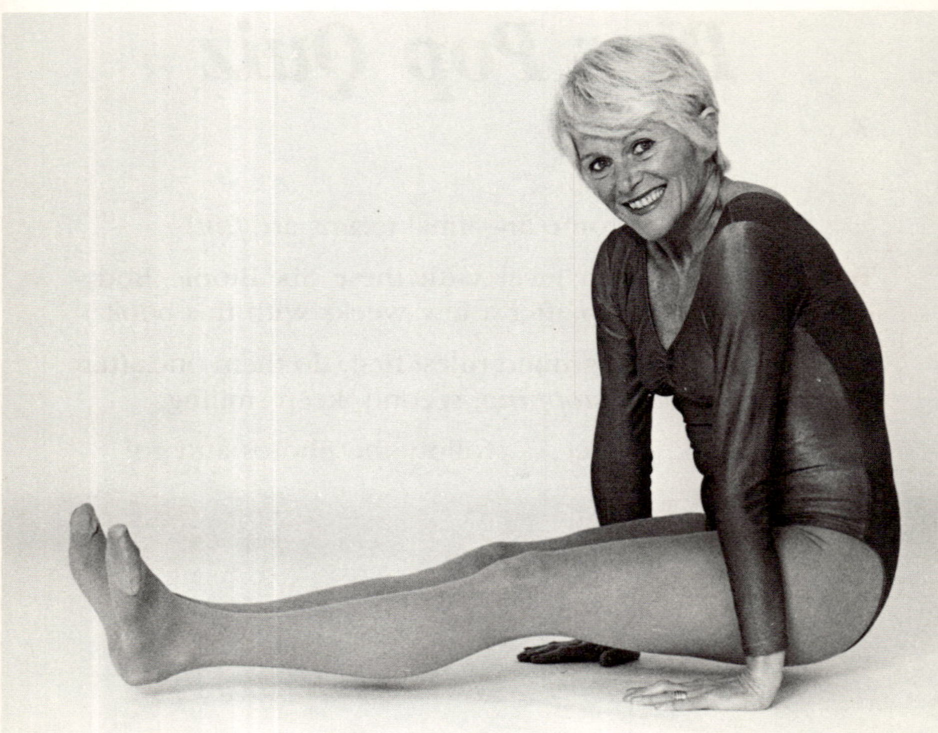

Sit on the floor, legs outstretched, palms on floor next to hips. Now lift your whole body and balance it on your hands for 60 seconds. (Okay, 15 seconds).

2 *Starfish Stretch*

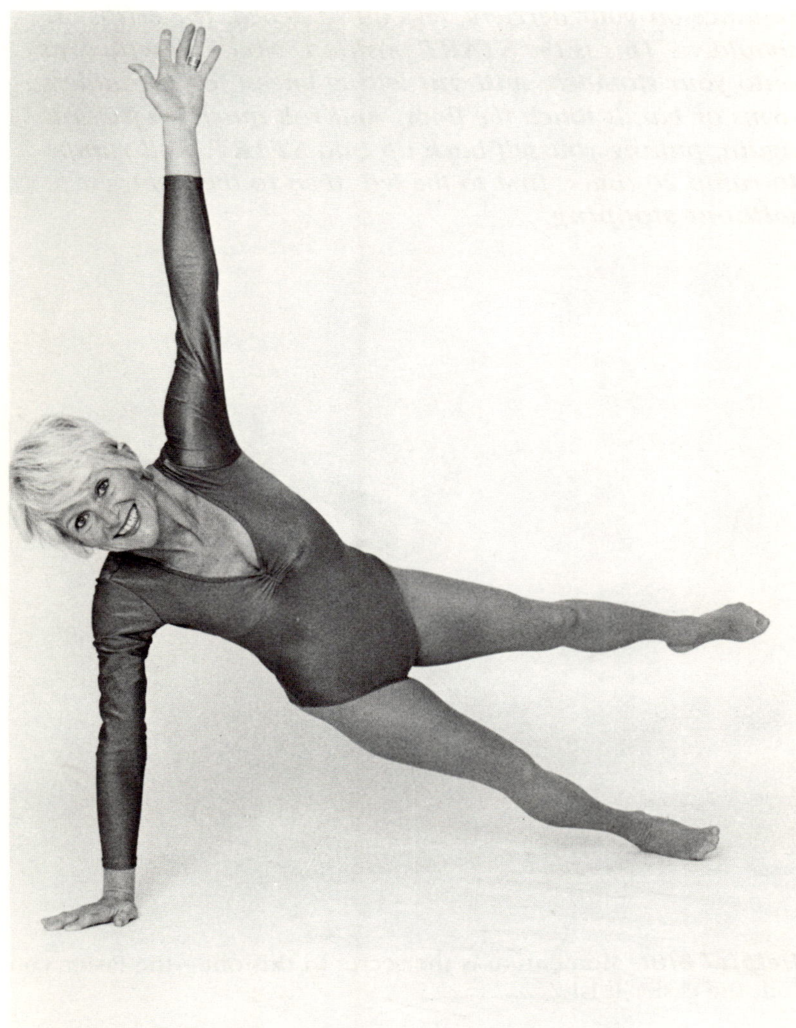

Balance on your right hand and the right side of your right foot; raise your left leg as high as you can and aim your left arm at the ceiling. HOLD for 60 seconds on each side.

3 *Sideways Rump-to-Rump Roll*

Balance on your derriere, legs outstretched, fingertips on shoulders. This is the ***START*** *position. Now roll leftwards onto your stomach,* ***without*** *letting knees, feet, shoulders, arms or hands touch the floor, and roll quickly leftwards again, pulling yourself back up into* ***START****. Roll rump-to-rump 20 times, first to the left, then to the right, etc.,* ***without stopping****.*

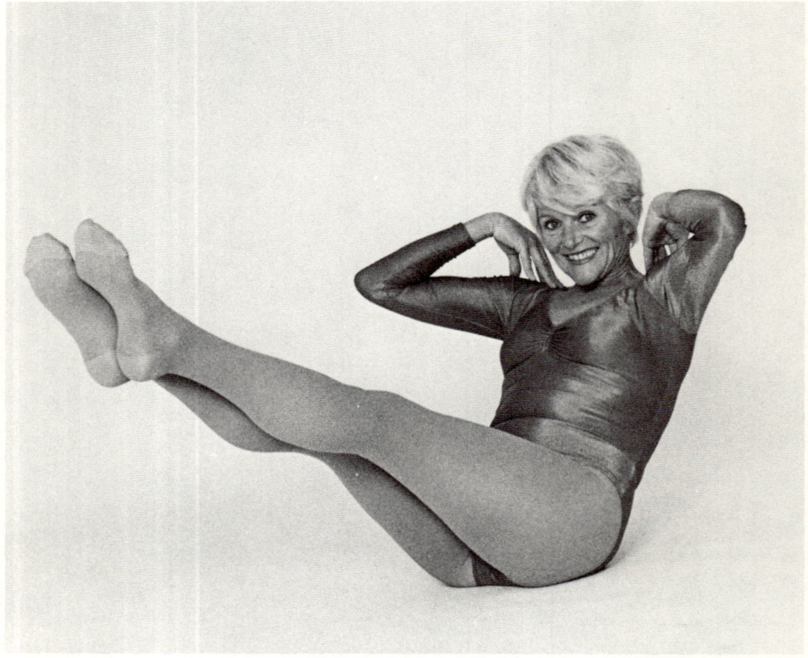

Helpful hint: Momentum is the secret to this one—the faster you roll, the easier it is!

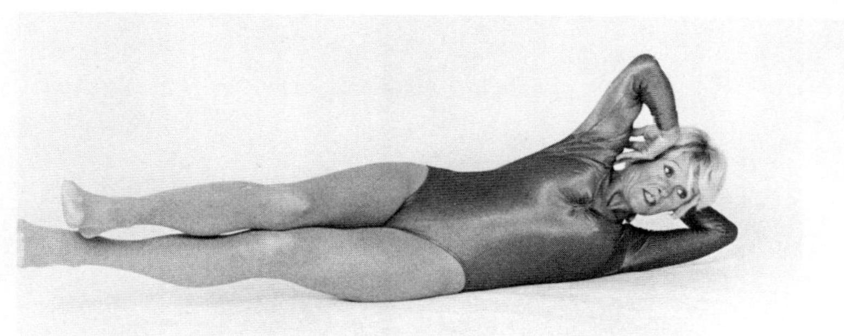

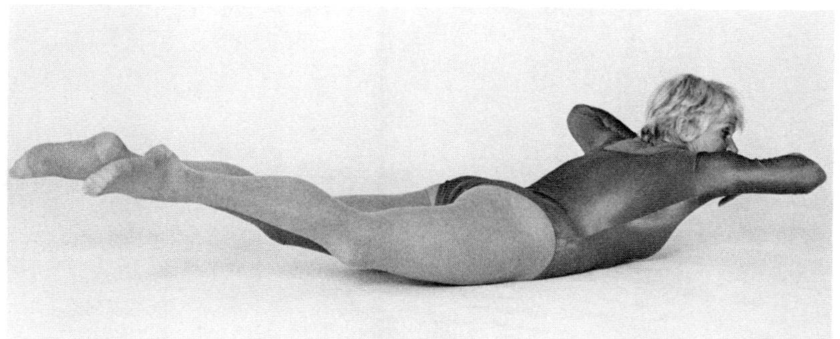

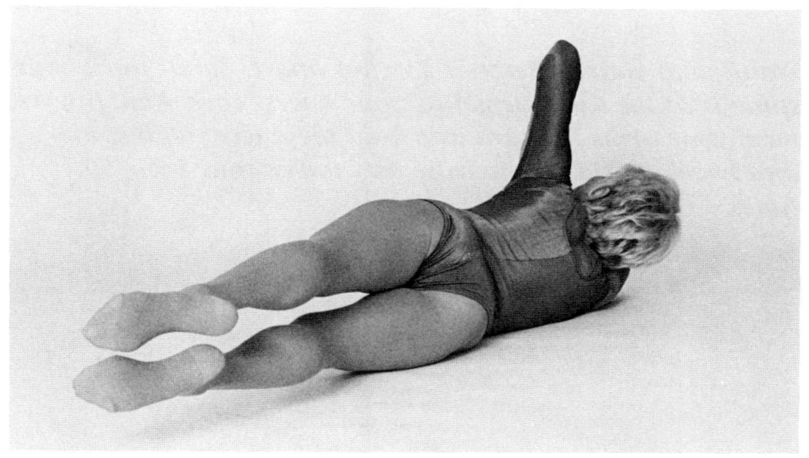

4 Heels-Up Squat

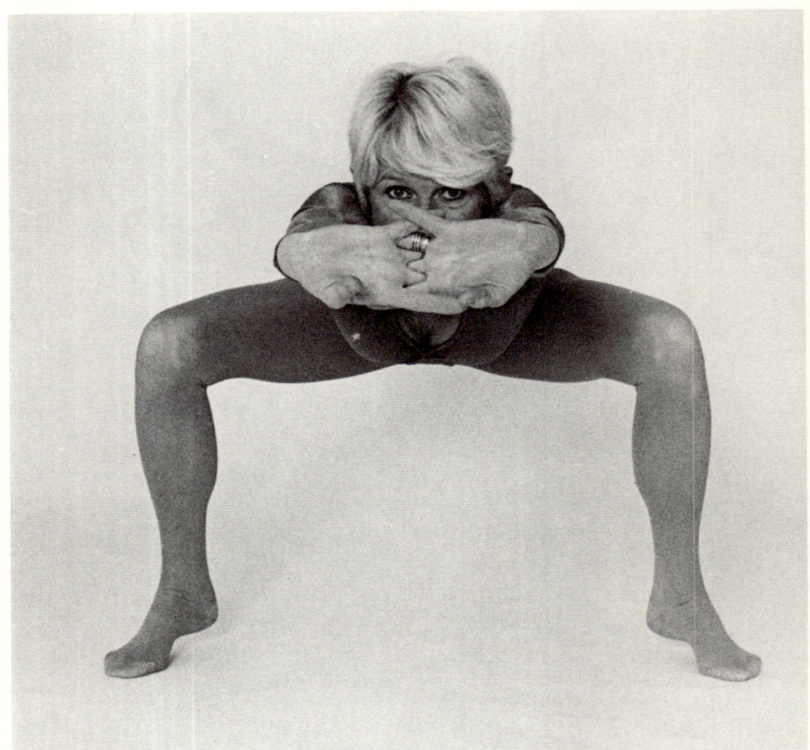

Stand with your feet about 2½ feet apart. Squat until your spine is at the same height as your knees. Lock your fingers, push your arms forward and hold them level with spine and knees. ***HOLD!*** *Now raise and lower your heels 50 times.*

5 Leg-Lift Headstand

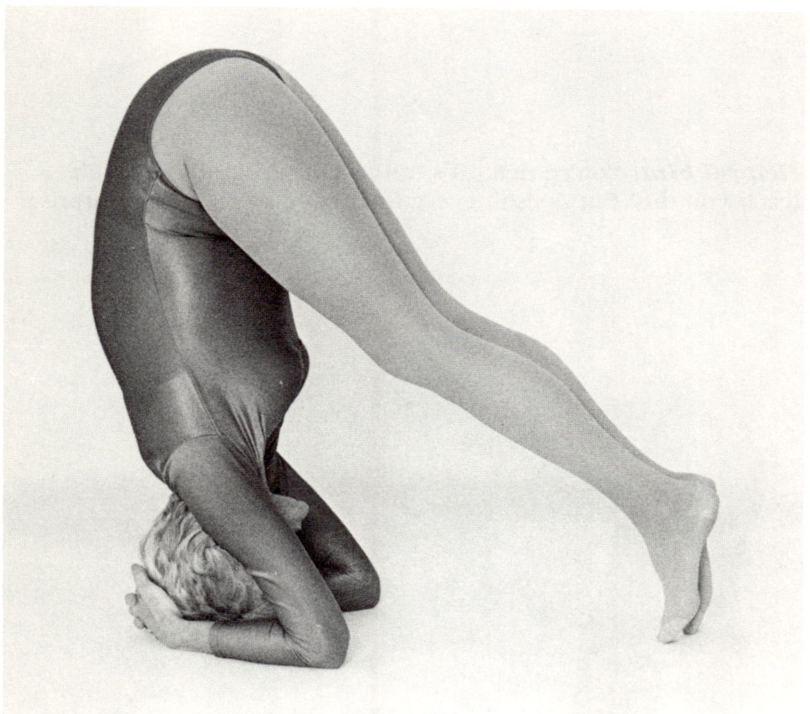

Start with toes on the floor, hands cupping head, weight on head and lower arms.

Helpful hint: You're right, it's not fair, it's Yoga and I didn't teach you this! But doesn't every final exam have a nasty surprise?

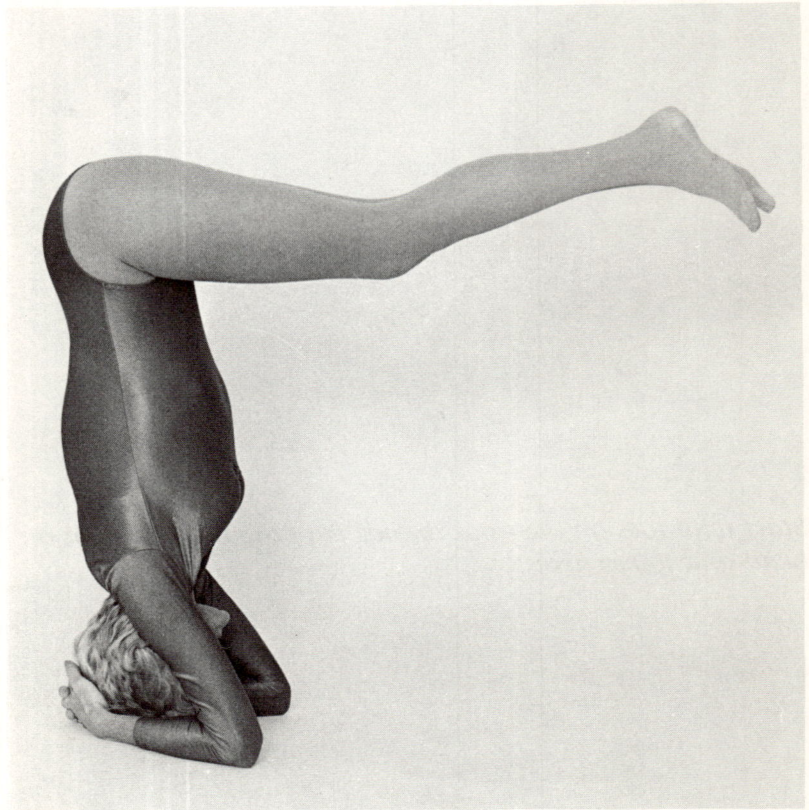

Now lift your legs, without bending them, from the floor to

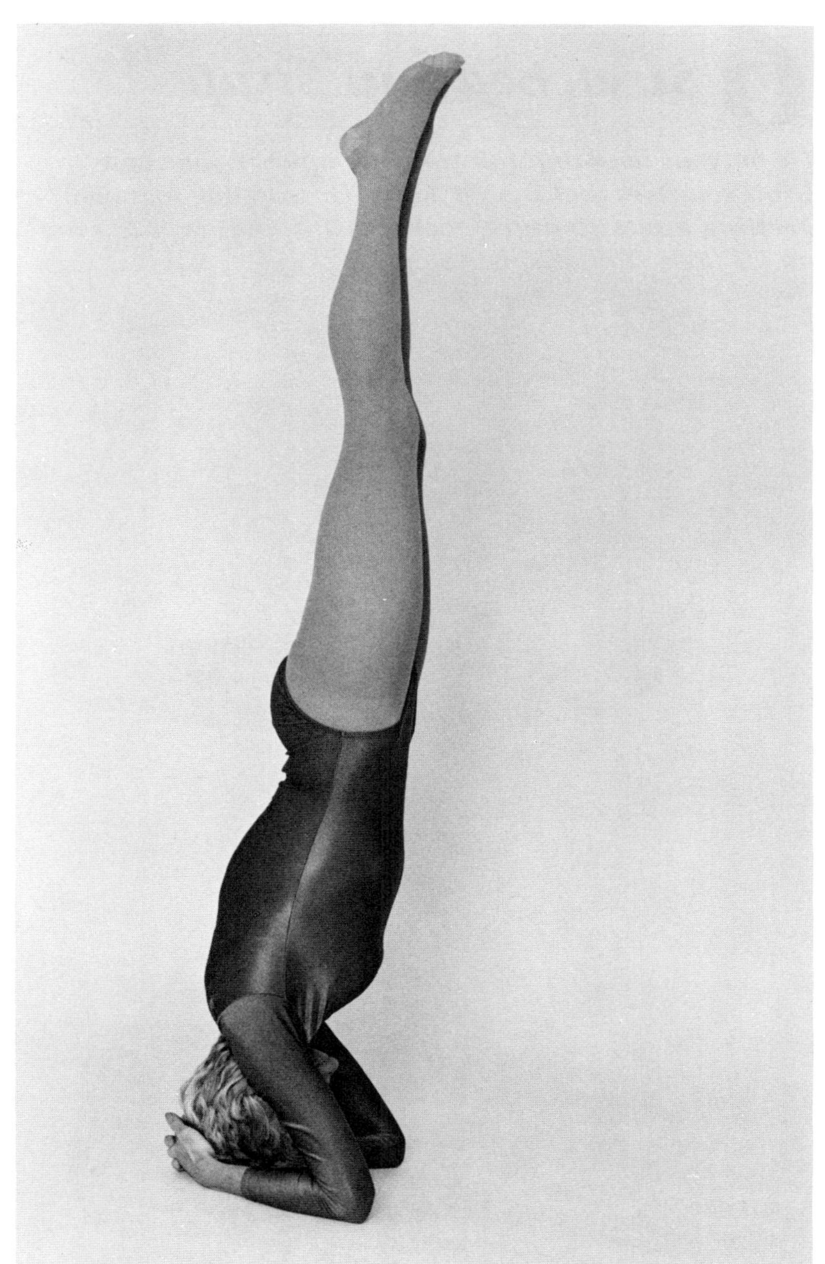

a straight upside-down position. Keeping your legs straight, return toes to the floor, touching down lightly without putting weight on toes. Perform lift 10 times without stopping.

6 *Stretched-Out Situp*

Lie on your back and roll your legs up over your nose. Grab your toes and **DON'T LET GO.** *Gripping toes and* ***keeping knees straight****, rock forward until your legs are on the floor. 20 times, non-stop.*

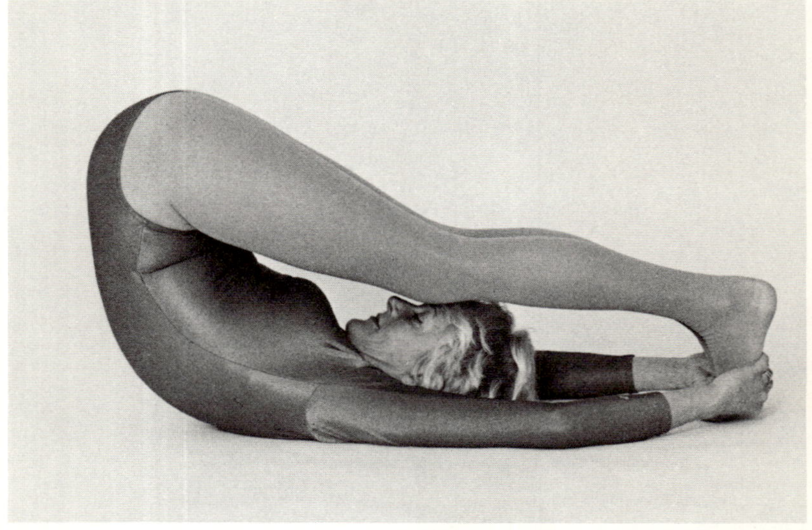

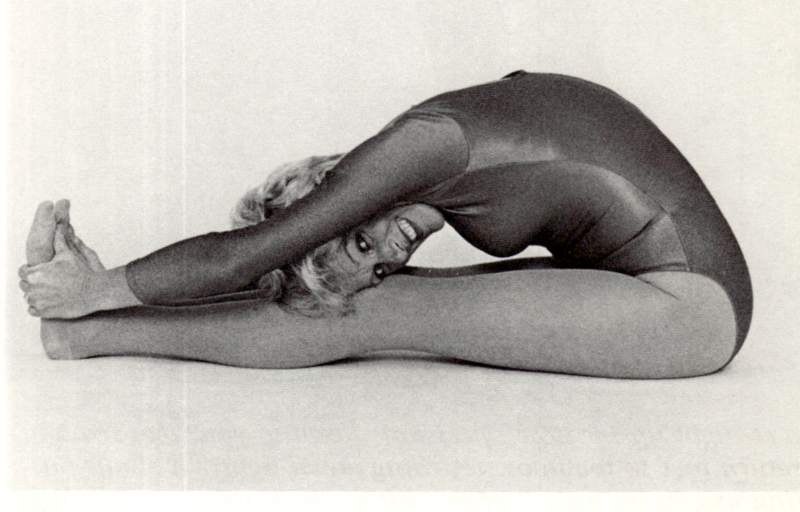

How to Score Yourself

If you only made it through one or two—
back to the Basic Eight with you!

3—Ho, hum.

4—Looking much better.

5—Looking *very impressive*.

All 6—Croix de Guerre, gold watch, and a lifetime job as defensive tackle on the team of your choice. You're **PERFECTION PLUS!**

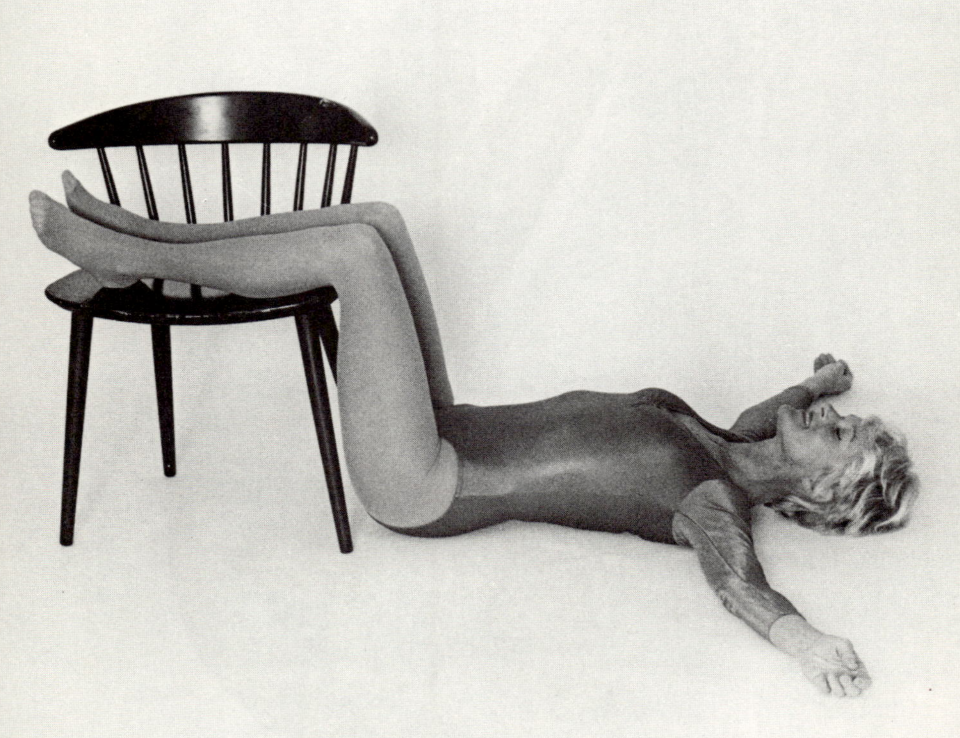

And if you can still move at all after this, turn the page for more treats.

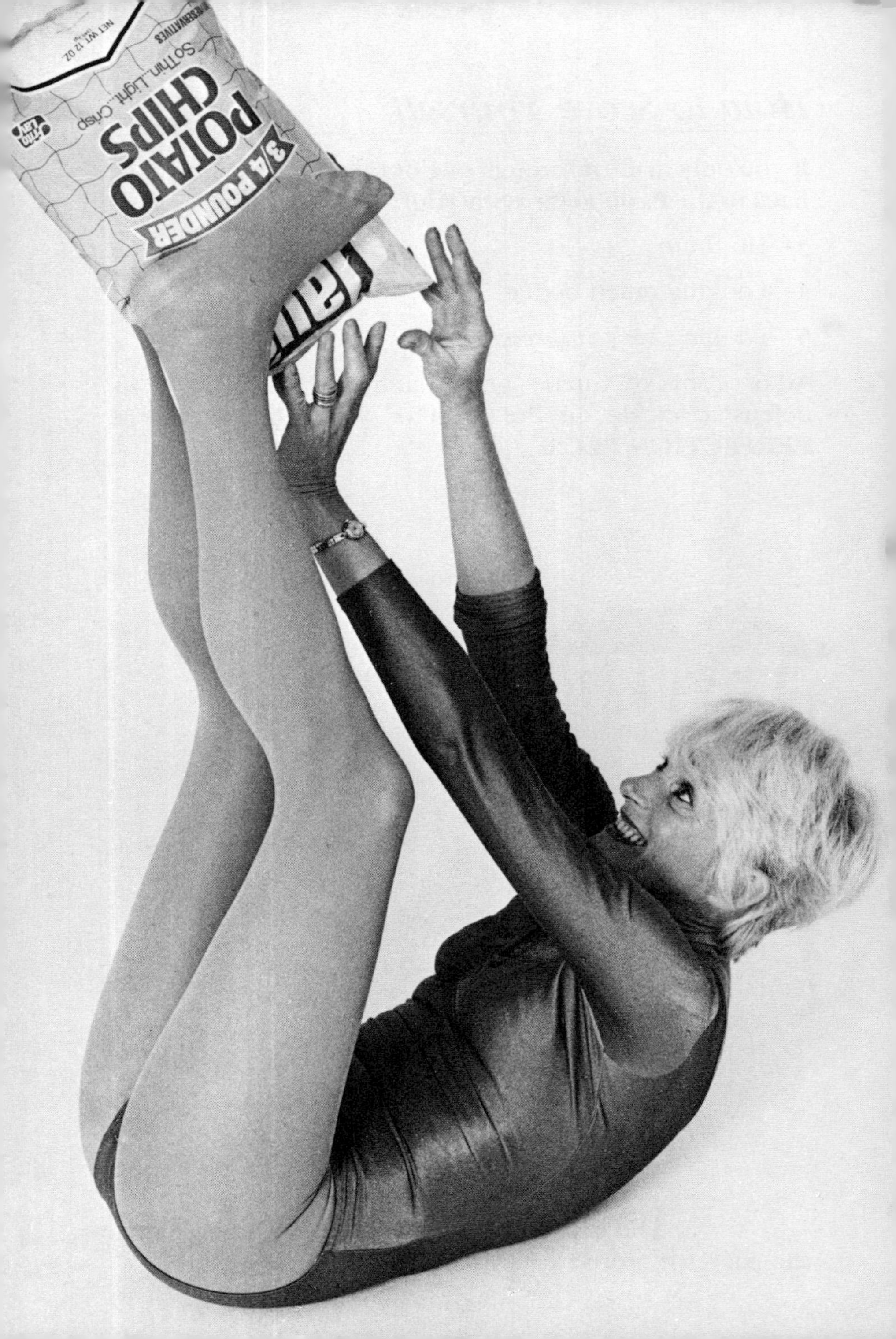
3/4 POUNDER
POTATO CHIPS
So Thin...Light...Crisp
NET WT. 12 OZ.

7 The Exerciser's Guide to Junk Food: Snacks, Wine, Beer, and Booze

Eat! Feed your face! Slurp it up and shovel it in—the grease, the sugar, the chips, the fudge, the booze, the burgers, the shakes, the fries, the cakes, the pies, the creamy, gloppy expense-account lunches—*anything you want!*

All you have to do is work it off—and you won't gain a millimeter. If soldiers and dancers and big time athletes can consume more than 6,000 calories a day and still be in top shape, why can't we all?

We can, if we follow a simple guide to balancing calorie intake with calorie burnoff.

The Balancing Act

1 piece pecan pie *(600 cals.)*	=	1 hour running 5.5 mph
1 piece cheesecake *(450 cals.)*	=	1 hour disco dancing, nonstop
1 serving eggplant parmigiana *(600 cals.)*	=	1 hour strenuous breast stroke, nonstop
1 quarter-pound hamburger with cheese *(514 cals.)*	=	1 hour jogging
3 pieces fried chicken *(900 cals.)*	=	1 hour horseback riding at full gallop *plus* 1 hour folk dancing
1 slice ice box cake *(300 cals.)*	=	1 hour golf, pulling cart
4 slices sausage pizza *(1,000 cals.)*	=	1 hour squash *plus* 1 hour handball
12 small French fries *(220 cals.)*	=	1 hour cleaning windows
1 small chocolate sundae with chocolate ice cream, chocolate sauce, and pecans *(500 cals.)*	=	1 hour vigorous ice skating
1 Danish *(275 cals.)*	=	1 hour cycling

The Balancing Act

1 serving macaroni and cheese *(430 cals.)*	=	1 hour tennis, vigorous singles
1 taco *(180 cals.)*	=	1 hour bowling
1 enchilada *(165 cals.)*	=	1 hour golf, in power cart
1 corned beef on rye with mustard *(540 cals.)*	=	1 hour downhill skiing
1 vanilla milkshake *(400 cals.)*	=	1 hour vigorous roller skating
1 12-oz. root beer *(150 cals.)*	=	1 hour slow dancing
3 glasses champagne *(270 cals.)*	=	1 hour pushing light power mower
3 glasses white or red wine *(240 cals.)*	=	1 hour gardening
1 12-oz beer *(150 cals.)*	=	1 hour ironing
2 daiquiris *(240 cals.)*	=	1 hour cleaning windows
2 Old Fashions *(260 cals.)*	=	1 hour mopping floors
2 vodka tonics *(450 cals.)*	=	1 hour water-skiing

Still Hungry? *EAT!* As long as you *KEEP MOVING*, all the equations are good!

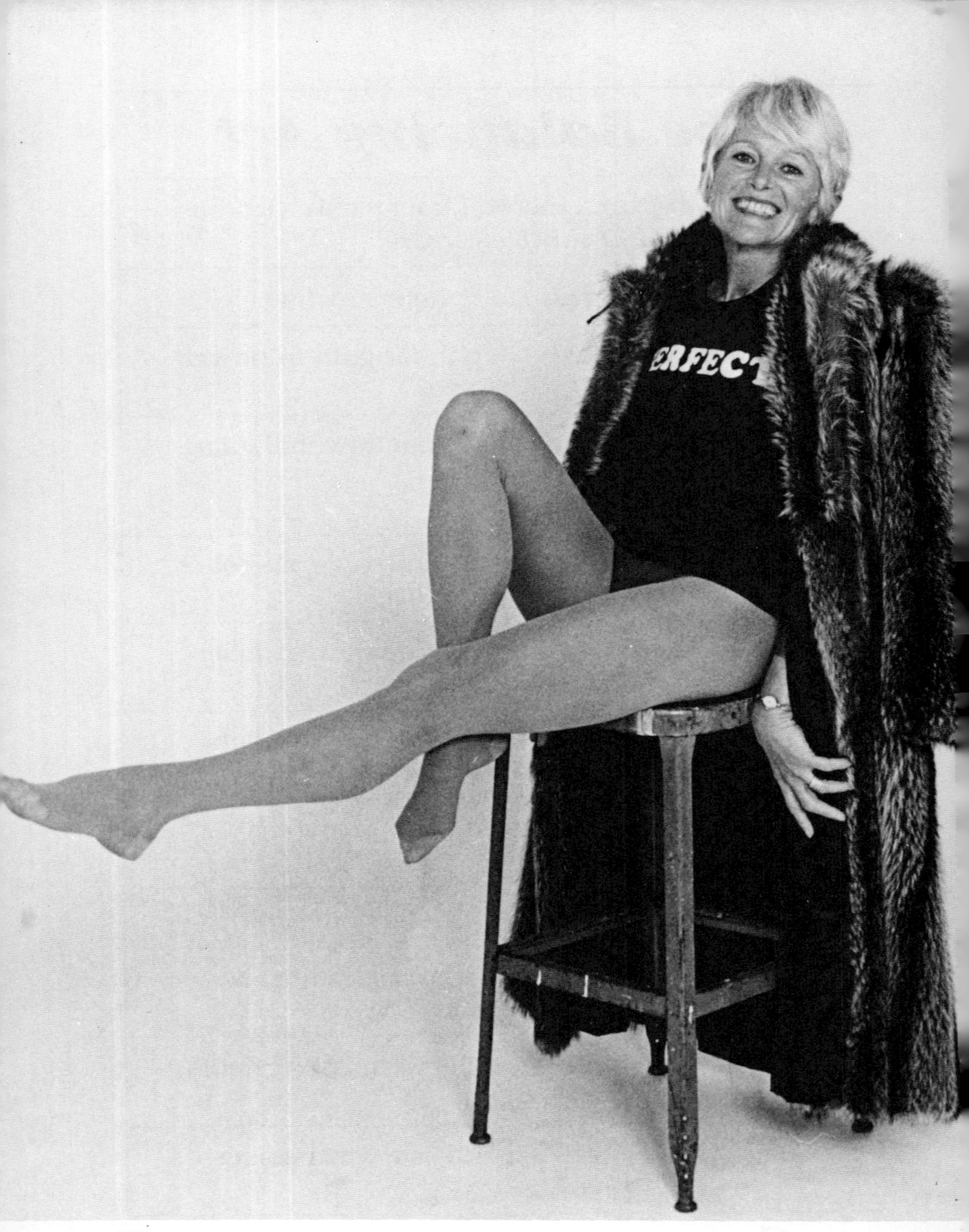